So, You Think
You Eat
Healthy
?

Linda Larrowe Bergersen

Nutrition Consultant, MS

Communications, BA

BOARD CERTIFIED IN HOLISTIC NUTRITION®
National Association of Nutrition Professionals (NANP) Member

This book contains the opinions and ideas of the author. It is intended to provide helpful general information, and not to replace advice of your personal health advisor.

A LifeTrends Publication

Palm Springs, CA

Printed in the United States

Printed by CreateSpace, An Amazon.com Company

Available from Amazon.com and other retail outlets

ISBN-13: 978-1493743896
ISBN-10: 1493743899

DEDICATION

I dedicate this to my husband,
the one person who has had
more faith in me and given more
inspiration than anyone. I could
not have completed this without
his spirit and ability to instill
confidence.

Thank you, Pat, for
inspiring the title.

Arianna,

Thank you for letting me contribute to your great HuffingtonPost.com

Linda

Table of Contents

To your health...

Introduction

We are drowning, people, in America's own design of convenience. The convenience of food, that is, and it is up to us individually and collectively to change that design.

Our design of convenience of course begins with our food source system involving food manufacturers, supermarkets and restaurants. Over the years these sources have all systematically come after our tastebuds, and created a fare that we desire, whether nutritional or not. Because of greed, competition and ignorance, the average American's internal system is out of balance, and being out of balance will only lead to disease. In fact, this convenience model has infiltrated other countries, and its damage of disease has already shown by increases in diabetes, heart disease, and obesity.

Our ever-expanding, industrialized society over the years has required the food industry to cater to the needs of those working outside the home, travelling, work, etc. Unfortunately it has gotten out of hand.

The companies that make food products, the restaurants that create exotic dishes both have had little regard for the nutritional value of the foods they offer the public. The supermarkets are eager to shelve whatever sells the best. We, the consumers, are dependent on what is convenient mostly because of time restraints. As convenience foods were developed and put on the shelves, people welcomed all they could get. Once fast foods were created, we were hooked on the convenience; sweet foods became sweeter and sweeter, thus making us addicts to sugar. We cannot mistake the worldwide sugar addiction as we see adults and children alike carrying around their drinks, daily.

Soon we were eating foods tainted with preservatives, dyes and trans fats, and not realizing it. Without complaints, the food industry continued to taint and degrade our food as they saw fit, primarily to make it sell. The longer it could stay on the shelf, the more they could sell; the prettier it looked, the more they could sell; the tastier it tasted, the more they could sell. And so it goes…yet at our expense.

These tactics continue today, but the public is now having second thoughts about these additives, and more and more are speaking up; but still not enough; we are still in the minority, as so many consumers are left in the dark about the degradation of our foods, and as those who would rather enjoy than complain turn a blind eye; it's these consumers who will unfortunately continue to develop the diabetes and heart disease or cancer.

There are many types of nutrition programs, diets and recommendations available from hundreds of doctors, nutritionists, dietitians, and fitness experts. Each professional has their own ideas of what is the best for maintaining health, so it is difficult to know what to follow or believe. In reading the history of foods, and seeing how the views of professionals have continually changed over the years, I'm open to thinking that much of what I and other professionals of today determine about foods could be viewed as all wrong twenty years from now.

Humans have been and are constantly adapting food intake according to social and environmental circumstances, and eating grains and fruit all year round is part of that evolution. A century ago, fruit was not available during the winter months in most parts of the world. What were the cavemen eating? Whatever they could find, depending on what part of the world they evolved.

We humans have done all right with ourselves – developing a highly intelligent mind, and living longer than the caveman could hope. One big problem in the modern world has been allowing those in charge of our foods to taint and alter them, and chip away at our progress of health. The average American's internal system is now out of balance.

When will we have fast-food restaurants offering true nutritional foods? When will we start entering a supermarket and not be immediately met with rows and rows of sugared drinks and junk food?

When will we stop believing what the television commercials tell us about their products in order to get us to buy?

When will the traditional medical community start believing in the value of nutrition for healing?

When will every person understand that *'you are what you eat?'* is actually true?

Understand that the intention of this book is to guide those who presently eat poorly into a world of better nutritional choices. It is not purported that the suggestions made within these pages are the ultimate *cure-all* answers to eating the most healthful foods of all time, but it is a start to get anyone on their way to more healthful eating. There are other books that advocate eating raw foods, and foods with funny names that can't be pronounced. No one is about to give up comfort foods so easily, and change their way of eating overnight, but as you learn what has happened to our food, and why it is important to change old habits, it will become easier to make new healthier choices, and they will become more tasty and satisfying. Each person can and will go about learning a better course of nutrition at his or her own pace.

It is touted from some that raw fruits and vegetables are the answer; or a vegan diet; or a Mediterranean diet. Some say don't eat grains because man did not eat them 20,000 years ago; and yet nuts are recommended, which possess many of the same anti-nutrients of grains. Some say grains possess nutrients we need. Some say don't eat meat; but yet without meat the needed nutrients of B12 and conjugated linoleic acid (CLA oil) are very difficult to acquire in the diet. Some say don't eat potatoes because either they're too starchy or too glycemic, or cause weight gain; and some say that 100 years ago our (natural) potato intake was twice as much as it is today, and today our cancer rate is twice as high as it was 100 years ago; and that there are tribes of people throughout the world that thrive on tubers as a staple in their diets and have no heart disease or obesity. There are fruits and vegetables that can be named that in one way or another can wreak havoc in certain people and not in others, which the average person is not aware of, as noted in Chapter nine. Taking this all in, there could be a problem with almost any food we eat today. If we were to listen to and follow all the professionals and their diet guidelines we would not be eating *eggs, meat, dairy, fruit, grains, beans, soy, salt, potatoes/tubers, oils/fats, sugars, starches.* So what would be left to eat? Vegetables...but not all of them.

Theories that have evolved from recent studies suggest that the start of man cooking foods and eating meat earlier in man's existence may have helped create larger brains in humans, which accelerated intelligence; some dispute this. Research reveals that humans who were meat eaters millions of years ago survived and evolved to homo sapiens, while the vegetarian man known as Paranthropus robustus disappeared from existence. Some say the possibility of eating grains may have had some influence on more intelligence as well; of course, 200 years ago, our grains were much more natural and healthful than they are today.

The art of healthful eating is an ongoing education, and at least recently there is a sense of a growing community on striving to determine the best diet we should have for bettering our health; this has a lot to do with the acceleration of media and the various avenues of communication in the 21st century. The more we can come together on solutions, especially between nutritionists, the medical community, and the food industry, the better off we will be as a society. As it stands today, we cannot win with eating manufactured, prepared foods.

The revelation for many that I want to make is that it is the refined foods that are not only hurting our health, they are what make us fat.

Right now it's all about satisfying ourselves. It seems our frenzy to satisfy our taste buds has overridden our need to *save* ourselves.

1

Chapter 1

Auto-Tune Your Body

Eat right, keep fit, and you'll still die. No matter what anyone tells you to do with your body, we all know that there is an inevitable end to our existence. Even by following rigorous nutritional diets, no one can dispute the fact that people still become sick with disease, some at younger ages than others, and even some of us who seem to treat our bodies with respect as opposed to those who abuse their bodies. Therefore, we must understand that there is more to this elusive thing called *perfect health* other than good nutritional foods and exercise.

However, eating right and exercising do play big roles in helping to prevent, alleviate or minimize what can happen to your body, whether it be inherited or acquired. Most importantly, proper health maintenance will afford you a better, more comfortable vehicle in which to travel this planet while you are here on earth. It could mean the difference between living twenty years longer (especially in cases of heart failure, cancer) or, more realistically, maybe only four or five. But most importantly, a nutritionally enhanced way of eating, along with exercise, will lead to a better quality of life in the years that we live.

After all, in essence, we *are* traveling on this planet in this vehicle we call a body. And traveling in it requires that we keep it fueled, keep it tuned, and keep good treads on the tires. And that is one reason why it is so appropriate to relate how we take care of our body to how we take care of our automobiles. In our society we seem to treat our automobiles with more care and respect than we do our own bodies, and we need to turn this around. For some reason the functioning of our bodies is so highly taken for granted…that is, until we grow older and are suddenly affronted with a catastrophic illness. Many look at common disorders as inevitable as age sets in, but that's not total reality. Our parts can be properly maintained, reconditioned, and cleaned out, just like those on a car, but many overlook this or don't believe that it can matter. It may be that we are more concerned about automobile parts than our own internal parts.

It is a luxury to have a car in good working condition at our whim to be free to travel anywhere at any time. We all know how confining and frustrating it would be to not have one, and only be able to rely on impersonal buses and trains. So the importance of getting to work on time and being able to run down to the store for bread on a rainy night lends us to be vigilant about the minor noise in the engine or the minor leak underneath, not to mention the intermittent maintenance we must do to prevent the horrific breakdown in the middle of nowhere.

People find it a necessary preventive routine to have regular oil changes on their car, or rotate tires and align the front-end. It is so important for everyone to maintain their automobile so it can get them around for an extended amount of time, but how about the body that gets you around more than anything? A question to pose to the ardent automobile owners (which is a vast majority in the United States), those who cherish their cars for their utility, freedom of travel and commuting, and of course for a statement of identity, is: why not treat your body as well as you treat your car? Isn't that a fair enough thing to do? *YOUR* vehicle needs to work before your automobile will be of any use to you. Why not clean your body out once a year? Why not keep it lubricated with the most adequate oil? Why not give it the proper fuel?

Nothing could be more important than monitoring the wellbeing of your body on a daily basis. Your car will run its best on the fuel made for its particular engine; the better the fuel, the better it runs; the higher the *octane*, the more energy you have.

Since traits that parents possess are frequently handed down to children, even those who haven't been raised by their parents, so can physical and/or physiological internal characteristics be inherited, such as genetic diseases, and so the predisposition of certain illnesses can be underlying to manifest at any time. But your internal defenses are what can keep most genetic predispositions at bay. It may well never manifest at all with the ultimate defense, and then one might never even know he possesses any certain threat within.

There is the huge contributing role that the mind plays in illness. Stress and trauma have negative consequences physically, and have been proven over and over, especially in heart attack cases.

Health is internal, external, physical, emotional and psychological. People invariably point to one thing, one cause, when they become ill, when instead people should search in each of these five areas to come to a more realistic reason. Any combination of the five variables can create an imbalance in the body, bring down the defenses, and bring about disease, as with skin cancer. A person who contracts skin cancer may point to the sun for the cause. But in reality, this type of thinking needs to change because it is not the sun alone that creates a cancer within the body.

Why is it that some people get skin cancer and some do not? We are all under the same sun. Our bodies are built with defenses, and some people have a better internal defense built up within than others; this defense is called our immune system. Without such things as white blood cells, antibodies, antioxidants, and T-cells circulating and patrolling within our body, we could not stay alive long. So as the drivers of our own vehicle, our body, we must do all we can to keep its defenses up against intruders such as viruses, bacteria, toxins, free radicals, etc. The harm done by these intruders entering our bodies is relevant to the amount of defenses stored within our bodies, our internal soldiers, so to speak. By building up our internal army, we can fight against disease. But for a person who smokes, drinks alcohol profusely, ingests large amounts of sugar, rancid or trans fats, and ingests processed foods, defenses will be destroyed on a daily basis by the adverse substances, and the body will be left very mildly guarded. Put sugar in your gas tank, and find out what happens.

It is a law that automobiles on the American highways be safe and non-polluting to society. As law-abiding citizens, we abide by the environmental and safety standards that we as a society adopt. If a car is seen on the road spewing out smoke from its tailpipe, it is automatically cited as a threat to the public's wellbeing, and ordered to be fixed.

Smoking

Smoking is an adverse term, with both automobiles and humans, only the big difference is that in the human body smoke is the cause of a disorder, and in the automobile, smoke is the effect. We put it in our bodies while cars are spewing it out...which indicates that the car is the more intelligent of the two. At least the car is trying to tell you something. By ingesting smoke and nicotine, the body tries to tell you something is wrong by aches, pains, coughing and such, until the emphysema or cancer shows up.

It is quite bewildering to hear individuals talk about eating healthfully and exercising while all along they continue to smoke. It is as if they are trying to fool others and/or themselves into thinking that they are actually being good to their bodies, and some even fool themselves into thinking that smoking has nothing to do with their physical problems. In fact, they are in total denial of what they are really doing to the functionality of their "engine", and what harm they are doing even to those around them.

Smokers are prescribed blood pressure medicines by doctors while they continue to smoke because they realize it's of no use to nag their patients about quitting. Every day smokers lose loved ones who have been fellow smokers and who pass away from related causes such as emphysema, lung cancer or heart disease. They see them burdened by the oxygen tanks; they see them struggle for a breath; or they anguish in the waiting room as they become admitted to the hospital because of a heart attack, but it doesn't jar them enough to quit the nasty habit and spare themselves and family the agony of the same diseases.

The toxins inhaled by smokers create a highly acidic environment where the cells in the body become altered and hindered. A person who smokes cigarettes has a risk of having a heart attack twice as much as an individual who does not smoke. When the nicotine enters the blood stream, blood platelets begin to clump up causing blood clots to develop. These clots bring about narrowed arteries either in the heart or the brain. When smokers have clogged arteries, results often include a heart attack, stroke, heart failure, or sudden death. Nicotine forces a smoker's blood pressure to rise. When inhaled, nicotine releases a hormone that requires the heart to work harder, increasing the heart rate, and blood circulation around the heart also becomes insufficient. The oxygen in the blood stream is replaced with carbon monoxide. The oxygen level declines significantly, not allowing enough oxygen to reach the heart or brain. Along with oxygen deprivation, the carbon monoxide attacking the heart is toxic and increases the amount of cholesterol that goes to the damage to help the problem, leading to clogged arteries. Tobacco sugars are formed on leaves as they are dried, and this sugar becomes a type of molecular glue when entering the bloodstream. When a smoker inhales, the sugars are absorbed in the lungs and attach to the walls of arteries, eventually blocking the arteries.

Cigarette smoking kills 390,000 Americans every year. 16% of all deaths that occur in the U.S. each year are the result of smoking. Pregnant women who smoke are putting their baby at risk for developing respiratory problems along with improper growth patterns. 4,000 babies die each year from complications brought about from their mother smoking during pregnancy.

Even the most passionate smoker would complain about seeing a car on the road spewing smoke from its tailpipe.

Fuel

The food we eat is our fuel that keeps us moving…and alive. Therefore, it makes perfect sense that the quality of foods we choose to put into our bodies does make a difference with the quality of our wellbeing and physical condition. If you drive a car with low octane, you will soon feel the lack of power in the engine.

Glucose is what fuels our bodies; it's our gasoline. Glucose is found in almost everything we eat: grains, sugars, vegetables, fruits, starches, carbohydrates. Carbohydrates convert to glucose, and that's where we get our energy, but the added refined sugars and flours we get in the typical American diet gives a higher octane than our engine can handle causing it to eventually let us down, and therefore we get into trouble with diabetes and such. It's the good carbohydrates that we run optimally on, like 100% whole grains and vegetables.

Oil Filter

Regular oil filter changes are considered mandatory to establish a long engine life, removing impurities. Our livers perform the same function as the oil filter, but never are we told of the necessity to clean our very own body filter. It too removes the impurities. And besides filtering, the liver has so many other functions that keep us alive; it distributes our nutrients; it aids our digestion; it produces our needed cholesterol, and so much more. It is the largest organ of our body (not including the skin), and in this day and age livers are constantly being abused and ignored. Removing toxins and the effects and overload of medications used today is a major job of the liver. Because of our heightened reliance on prescription drugs today, and heavy societal use of recreational drugs, tobacco and alcohol, our livers are extremely overworked; enough that they can't keep up with their job of trying to keep us well. Reaching an overload, and the liver shuts down. Simple liver cleansing foods include lemons, watermelon and asparagus.

Carburetor

The function of the carburetor is controlling the air/fuel mixture going to the automobile engine. The carburetor breathes life into the engine, and human lungs breathe life into the body. Carburetors become dirty from dirty air filters; lungs can become polluted from smog, chemicals, bacteria, and the bright idea of sucking smoke directly into them. Lungs and liver are both involved in excretion of impurities, but the more junk that goes in, the harder it is to filter out. This is why exercise is so important. Exerting muscles to move needed oxygen to every cell of the body helps in the filtering of the air/fuel mixture going to our engine.

Gas Pedal

The speedometer on the dashboard of cars may go as high as 200 miles per hour, normally around 120 mph, yet we never drive that fast. The laws make us drive way below that, keeping us from having excessive amounts of accidents that would occur otherwise. And so we should have a similar unwritten law pertaining to the burners on our stoves. Fewer foods should be cooked, and more raw foods eaten. And the foods we do cook should never be cooked above the 'medium' setting, and most should never be cooked above 'low'. Most foods cook quite well at the 'low' setting.

Many feel that cooking our fuel (food) is a huge demise to our wellbeing. All foods are full of natural enzymes whose main functions are to self-digest the foods that enter our bodies; they are giving our body the gift of aiding our digestion. The more foods we cook, the less aid we get, and the more our bodies must work harder to take in the fuel.

Besides the loss of enzymes in cooking, there are several toxic elements created in cooking. This is especially important for cooking such foods as eggs and starchy foods like potatoes. Omega 3 content can become oxidized; acrylamide can form in foods that have been "browned". Browning meats is an unnecessary procedure. The extreme direct high heat exposure adds toxins to the food; meats will cook perfectly fine without the step of 'browning' it. (See chapter 6, *Cooking Heat*.)

Cooking at low temperatures is an important consideration in the transition to better, healthier eating habits, as is consuming more raw foods.

"In order to change we must be sick and tired of being sick and tired"

~ Author Unknown

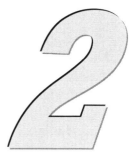

Chapter 2

Balance is What It's All About
The Body Works FOR Us, Not Against

There are checks and balances constantly going on naturally throughout the body unnoticed by us as we go through our daily lives. The functions of our bodies are so precisely orchestrated, far more than any of us realize. We take for granted how our bodies work - working at maintaining the balance we need to stay alive and healthy – systematically on its own. Think of how we make that step up a staircase without even thinking about it. Our foot goes up and lands precisely on the step. The same types of automatic functions are going on inside our bodies. The food is eaten and is automatically digested and disseminated to points within that are waiting to use the nutritional parts.

Not many realize that when we overload our system with a substance, signals are sent to the brain to release certain minerals or peptides for compensation. When we drink too much alcohol, which depletes (or kills) certain nutrients, signals are sent to release substances such as calcium to make up for the loss; the body will literally take it from the bones to make up for the loss due to alcohol or soft drink consumption. It is absolutely amazing the dynamics playing within our bodies on an ongoing basis. It's like having a battalion of soldiers and workers inside, always on guard, always working, always repairing, always defending. If something's not working right within us, on the most part, it is not perpetrated by our body, but rather mostly by something we have done to it or ingested.

Then something becomes out of balance. Being out of balance means that we are on the path to disease. As with the tires on the car; when the car is out of alignment, the tires can wear improperly, thus one tire may be in need of replacement. And if that isn't replaced, then other tires could be affected. And so it goes with your body. There may be many steps to getting to the origin of any problem within the body, and all that we find need to be corrected and rebalanced.

Most of us have the belief that our bodies will just break down eventually on their own, and nothing to do with what we've contributed. Well, of course there is the inevitable, but it does not have to happen sooner than later, and does not have to happen with so much pain and disability. Our mind and what it chooses to put into the body, and also the hidden additives or toxins that we are unaware of, have created the disorder.

Balance is created or corrected by foods you eat, detoxification and health practices you uphold. The human body is a self-regulated, self-defended, initially, innately balanced piece of machinery. It is up to the mind that resides in it, to maintain that balance, and, ironically, that mind itself is driven by what it is fed. Like the chicken and the egg, does the mind drive the food, or does the food drive the mind?

A depressed person cares little about having a healthy body, because the mind is not in a healthy state. On the other hand, not eating properly as well as not fortifying the system with the proper nutrients could very well be a major contributor to depression. If a person is positive and eager to keep their body in tune, then they will be positive and eager about taking notice at every meal of what they are putting into their system.

It comes down to wanting to help your self. We each have the required information in our heads to realize the path that brought us to a certain health dilemma. The doctor can't unlock your brain and follow that path precisely. It takes effort to retrack your steps, but this effort could prove to be more beneficial than having a doctor to try and figure it out.

Being overweight, having acid reflux, or just having a headache signals that the body is out of balance in some way, and the main reason the body gets diseased is because of the wrong things going into it and the disruption of the natural environment it was meant to live in.

As it is, there are many different theories, different calculations, when it comes to nutrition. You may have noticed that one year you are told something is good for you, and the next it is not. On the most part, it is the media that steers people wrong by getting their information from misinformed sources, and not from the nutritionists, the researchers who, over the years, have had consistent figures and information that unfortunately has not been unearthed or disseminated to the public. The media instead seems to rely more on the information of the pharmaceutical industry. The nutrition community has tended to be subdued, keep a low profile, since over the decades they have been blasted by the naysayers, the powerful pharmaceutical companies, the medical community, and those who cannot comprehend the body's natural ability to heal. The media seems to end up with facts that have evolved from those entities that want to suppress the feasibility and use of natural foods as well as nutritional supplements.

All one needs to do is read a little explanation of just one of the millions of processes that are going on within you every second of every day; you don't have to understand it, but it just gives an interesting picture:

> "Glucose in the bloodstream diffuses into the cytoplasm and is locked there by phosphorylation. A glucose molecule is then rearranged slightly to fructose and phosphorylated again to fructose diphosphate. These steps actually require energy, in the form of two ATPs per glucose. The fructose is then cleaved to yield two glyceraldehyde phosphates (GPs). In the next steps, energy is finally released, in the form of two ATPs and two NADHs, as the GPs are oxidized to phosphoglyc-erates." *(Muscle Physiology Laboratory, University of California, San Diego, http://muscle.ucsd.edu/musintro/glucose.shtml)*

This sounds like rocket science, but reading between and around all of the long, scientific names, a picture presents itself of the glucose sequence naturally taking place in our body, by no means of our own manipulation; by no effort on our part.

The human body is an amazing self-sufficient mechanism; it comes equipped with all the bells and whistles to keep its self aligned and running well. It needs and deserves the fuel it was meant to have; it needs the protection of a healthy natural environment it was meant to live in. Eating the right foods is so important to this balance.

Balance is the key to anything; the key to the universe and all within it. If one planet's orbit becomes out of sync, then life on earth is threatened. If one of the sparkplugs in the car goes bad, then the car will not perform properly. And, yes, there must be a balance within the body to keep it running smoothly.

One of the most important balances within the body is pH – the balance of alkalinity and acidity. Our bodies are naturally programmed to maintain this balance, and make a constant effort, but if the person is consistently eating acidic foods day by day, meal by meal, the body's efforts will be exhausted. The foods we eat are the predominant regulator of the pH. Certain foods create alkalinity and certain other foods create acidity. Too much of one of these will make a person become sick, diseased, and possibly die. The optimum Ph balance within the body that will maintain a healthful state consists of 80% alkaline and 20% acid. If the reverse of this were the case, disease would surely find its way to take over, creating havoc to the system. A diet predominantly built on hamburgers, hot dogs, fried foods, refined flours, refined sugars, and desserts raises the acidity level in the body tremendously; these foods are all acid, and the avoidance of fresh fruits and vegetables, which are mostly alkaline, surely will put the system out of balance.

Anything that threatens the balance of the body has disease-producing potential. Symptoms are red flags, signals of unrest in the body. They can be headaches, weight gain or heart palpitations. Any treatment designed to merely suppress unpleasant symptoms diminishes the body's ability to protect itself. The aspirin is one example.

It's known that Hippocrates (400 BC) prescribed a powder made from the willow tree for reducing fever and pain, and it was used in China and Europe continually through the centuries. The substance in the willow tree that proved to be of benefit was salicin, and that is what drug companies extracted in order to produce a product that would come to be called aspirin; yet another drug with origins of natural plants. Taking one ingredient from a living plant, concentrating it, and administering to a human does not always have the same results as the whole natural source. That one ingredient can cause havoc to the body merely because it does not have its balancing natural adjunct ingredients to make it work right. The aspirin as it is today affects the natural enzymes in our body, among other things. Relieving pain with aspirin, ibuprofen or acetaminophen may have you feeling better, but it is not healing whatever is going on inside that caused the pain in the first place. Fevers are actually created by the body to aid in destroying whatever invader is causing problems. On top of it, these substances are toxic; the body never asked for this type of help.

Our bodies are well-tuned mechanisms. Before disease is apparent, the body internally is juggling and attempting to realign itself through its own regenerative mechanisms at the cellular level. All this maintenance takes place every minute of every day without us even aware of it. In fact, as our bodies conduct constant maintenance, in essence our bodies are working toward rejuvenation daily; we can be a newer person every day, just as our skin cells are shed and new ones arise. It is when the body has reached the point where it can no longer juggle on the molecular level to try to bring things back into balance that symptoms become evident.

The major culprits of balance disruption in our bodies

There is too much time and emphasis put on calories, glycemic load, and particular foods such as bananas because they contribute too much sugar; or beef because it is too fatty; or eggs because they have too much cholesterol. Just think whole, real food. As long as you can detect what a whole, real food is, it's much easier to keep yourself out of harm's way.

The main sources of disease and obesity are two things, administered deliberately or unsuspectingly: food and chemicals. Here are just some of the most prevalent culprits:

Through foods/water:

> Pesticides on or in foods we eat
> Plastics, contaminating foods and water
> Chlorine, fluoride in water
> Teflon cookware leakage
> Altered foods

External sources:

> Prescription drugs
> Over-the-counter drugs
> Recreational drugs
> Cigarettes
> Smog
> Vaccinations
> Tooth fillings
> Cleaning products
> Anti-bacterial soaps
> Dyes in beauty products/lotions
> Electromagnetic radiation *(cell phones, electrical wires, x-rays, etc.)*

The more exposed to these elements, the more chance there is of getting sick. I do not want to discount the external sources, but mainly want to address the altering of foods over the decades as a prominent reason for our decline in health. Because we eat breads without bran and germ, because we drink milk that has been pasteurized and homogenized, because we put refined sugared water in our arteries daily, is why we are sick and overweight. The person who eats the most of these altered foods will be the one more likely to become sick and/or overweight.

Our bodies need all of the components of food: carbohydrates (glucose/natural sugars/starch), protein and fat/oil. If we were to eliminate or drastically reduce one of these, our system would then become out of balance because of it. There is an optimum ratio of these, which it seems has not been properly established as yet because there are so many professional health figures that keep going around and around about what is best for us. The balance of these could keep us in great health, and deter weight gain, as long as all the refined products of any of the main components are totally avoided.

It's not about counting calories, or we could have a candy bar for breakfast, lunch and dinner, and be within our allotted amount. It's not about 'low carb' because all fruits and vegetables are carbohydrate, and we need an abundance. It's not about the glycemic load, or we should be ingesting more ice cream (*1/2 cup =68gl*) than sweet potatoes (*1/2 cup =161gl*).

As for counting calories, it is a one hundred year old idea that really does not work. It does not work in losing weight because the real factor behind losing weight and being healthy at the same time is the type of food that is eaten, the right type of calories.

It turns out there are differences in calories if food is fermented, cooked or eaten raw. Calories are used up depending on the process of digestion needed by different types of foods. How foods have been grown can affect calorie usage, as well as how much the food has been processed. And lastly, different body types have different metabolic actions in relationship to calories. Counting calories is just another waste of time and effort when the time and effort could be placed on making sure the best types of foods are used as our fuel.

Sugar/Sweeteners/Glucose

The major disruption to our nutritional balance is our addiction to sugar, and how we've manipulated foods in order to get as much as possible. Mother's milk contains its natural sugar, and there is nothing but goodness coming from it. That is our first taste of sweetness, even though it's there to nourish, and not just to satisfy. Unfortunately, too high a percentage of women now feed their babies a poor substitute called formula. All that is included is unnatural, manmade. The sweetness mostly comes from corn maltodextrin; some brands add sucrose. The addiction could be starting here, and continues with sugars added to many brands of baby foods, and so on.

Glucose is the fuel we require to function, but over the centuries we have discovered the art of obtaining as much sugar as we desire; its effect on our brain is overwhelmingly satisfying.

When we bite into a piece of fruit, we get sweetness. But of course we don't bite into an agave plant or maple tree because getting any sugar is a difficult process. We have learned that these plants contain sweet substances, and we have learned how to extract them, and have learned how to even improve or exaggerate the taste. But in doing so, we've created the imbalance in those substances, which in turn create an imbalance in our internal system because they are not what our bodies were designed to process.

Even a substance that has been extracted is considered a processed food because you are eating just a part of that food, not every part as a whole. This includes such things as coconut sugar and olive oil. To truly have the whole food you must eat the coconut flesh or the olives. Some extracted substances, such as expeller-pressed oils, have shown anti-inflammatory effects, but the amount of highly processed oils and such must be kept at a minimum to achieve homeostasis (*the state at which a body has a healthy balance*).

Fructose

Research into fructose is increasing because of its current overuse as an additive to foods that began several decades ago. The many forms of extracted fructose, including high fructose corn syrup, are used in energy bars, ketchup, bakery goods, soft drinks and energy drinks. Its effects on the human body are currently being studied extensively as it is suspected as a factor in the nation's rise in obesity and disease. We devour five times more fructose than we did a hundred years ago because of its inclusion in so many foods. Once extracted and processed, being without fiber, etc., its value to the human system is changed. The fructose by itself and the fructose contained in its natural form within foods are two different things.

Fructose is a natural component in fruits, but most people do not realize that it is inherent in some vegetables and other foods. Apples have one of the highest amounts of natural fructose with 10,000 mg in one medium apple, and in perspective, a cup of cabbage contains 1300 mg. Eating two apples is almost as much fructose in a can of cola. But are we to assume that eating apples is as bad as drinking a can of coke? It is shown that in Greece, where part of their normal diet includes high fructose fruits such dates and honey, the triglyceride rates are quite low.

Fructose is mainly processed in the liver. The more fructose the more pressure on the liver, as well as increase triglycerides. While it is postulated that fructose does damage to our system, fructose does not raise blood sugar levels. Diabetics are told to eat apples because foods with a high amount of fructose do not spike blood sugar. So, are we doing them harm in this respect? And the same is true of agave, the high fructose sweetener; however, agave, unlike the apple, is highly processed, and that is the factor in leading to trouble.

On one hand, consuming fructose will not cause blood sugar spikes, but high consumption of fructose does contribute to insulin resistance, leading to diabetes. Yes, as an extracted substance used abundantly as an additive, it can cause harm. Drinking fruit juice is also a very high contributor of fructose because it is an extracted substance without fiber, apple juice having the highest. It is the whole accompaniment of contents in fruits and vegetables, such as fiber, enzymes and phytonutrients that help keep the natural sugars from reaping harm.

It is now being considered that eating too much fruit could have these same side effects, but in these times of too much refined sugars, especially fructose, it seems unfair to include natural fruit in the blame. I question whether to buy into a current recommendation of not eating fruit or certain fruits because the fructose content is high. For so very long we have eaten fruits and vegetables without regard to fructose, and now all of a sudden the apple turns out to be an actual forbidden fruit? From my perspective, it comes back to balance. If we were to include apples in a daily balanced diet of vegetables, grains, starches, protein and fat, without consuming any processed foods, there is no need for counting fructose amounts, as well as calories, carbs, or fats.

Fruit has always been considered *nature's perfect food*. As with the apple, if it contains a high amount of fructose, it is there for a reason, as part of that apple's balance of nutrients that make it an apple...naturally; after all, as it has been said, "an apple a day keeps the doctor away." Of course, if we were to eat apples morning, noon and night, and relied on fruit as our staple and bulk of our diet, it would definitely cause an imbalance that triggers disease.

Most fruits and vegetables contain approximately half fructose and half glucose, so there is really no way to eliminate the natural fructose from our diet unless you eliminated so many natural foods that have been deemed good for you for so very long. Fructose is a natural, safe sugar as long as it stays intact with the whole food.

A balanced body will require a person to include a balance of fruit, vegetables, grains, protein and fat, and not the elimination of this food or that food just because it has a high glycemic load, or high fat content, etc. It comes down to the factors behind how that food was made, manipulated or grown. It has to do with how much of that food is eaten in a day as opposed to all the other food groups: fruits, vegetables, grains, fats and protein. Are steaks eaten at every meal? Was the steer and cow fed corn and soy, or was it grass-fed? Is the bread 100% whole grain without sugar? Including an apple or banana every day in the diet gives fiber, vitamins, minerals and phytonutrients; in contrast, the daily diet soda is most definitely an anti-nutrient food...ingredients that do nothing except antagonize the path to health.

Certainly, with eating fruit, it matters if a person is diabetic. If a person has diabetes, it means they have eaten a constant diet over time of processed foods. That person would need to eliminate all sugars, including fruit and refined foods, while enforcing a strict natural, whole foods diet void of processed foods to get back into balance. Once the body is in balance, once the person discontinues the processed diet, and invariably consumes natural foods in a balanced manner, Type 2 diabetes will most likely disappear.

We were meant to eat fruits and vegetables, and each with their unique differences offers us a variety of micronutrients that ward off disease.

Since sugar is such a huge facet in our lives, I've included below a chart listing all the main popular sugars. *(Artificial sweeteners are not listed since they should never be used, as they are off the chart with their processing and chemical usage.)*

This chart shows how much processing they've endured, if they are acidic to the body or alkaline, etc. These are the factors most important to our health. Sugars are put into four categories of processing, from natural to extreme, usually through these methods:

Natural	*- whole form, ground or dried*
Extracted	*- liquid taken out, dried*
Minimal	*- extracted, heated/boiled*
Moderate	*- extracted, filtered, enzymatic breakdown, some processing, boiled*
Extreme	*- use of chemical processing, additives or lime, through multiple stages, bleaching*

In reviewing this chart, here are some things to consider:

- It's more healthful to eat the natural or lesser processed sugar
- Alkaline sugars are preferred
- Glycemic load is primarily a concern for diabetics and those who eat a high processed diet
- Comparable sweetness is necessary to know for recipes

Now you have a better picture of what sugar additive you may prefer.

Common Processed Sugars

SUGAR	PROCESS	FRUCTOSE/ GLUCOSE Ratio	pH	GLYCEMIC LOAD	SWEETNESS Compared to Table Sugar
Table Sugar	Extreme	50%/50%	Acid	HIGH	--
Brown Sugar	Extreme	50%/50%	Acid	HIGH	Same
Agave	Extreme	60-90%/ 10-40%	Acid	LOW	133%
HFCS	Extreme	55%90%/ 10%-45%	Acid	HIGH	Same
Dextrose	Extreme	-- / 100%	Neutral	HIGH	70%
Molasses	Moderate	50%/50%	Alkaline	MEDIUM	150%
Luo Han	Moderate	50%/50%	Alkaline	0	250%
Stevia	Moderate	--	Alkaline	0	300%
Brown Rice Syrup	Minimal	30%/30% 40%Maltose	Acid	HIGH	75%
Maple Syrup	Minimal	60%/40%	Acid	MEDIUM	133%
Sorghum Syrup	Minimal	50%/50%	Acid	MEDIUM	165%
Turbinado/ 'Raw sugar'	Minimal	50%/50%	Acid	MEDIUM	Same
Honey	Minimal	40%/30%	Acid	HIGH	150%
Erythritol	Minimal	--	Alkaline	0	70%
Xylitol	Minimal	from xylose	Alkaline	LOW	Same
Sucanat raw sugar	Extracted	50%/50%	Alkaline	LOW	Same
Coconut sugar	Extracted	48%/50%	Alkaline	LOW	90%
Stevia Green	Natural	--	Alkaline	0	300%
Date sugar	Natural	50%/50%	Alkaline	HIGH	130%
Raw Honey	Natural	50%/50%	Alkaline	MEDIUM	150%

** *Many brands of sweeteners, no matter the source, sometimes combine other lesser quality forms of sugars with theirs; always read the ingredients. You may not be getting what you think, including processed sugar.*

3

Chapter 3

What Were They Thinking?

Over the last 200 years our foods have been degraded, tainted and compromised by refinement, chemicals and processing. We know that before all this began, people were dying at a very early age. Our life expectancy has doubled in the last 200 years, despite the degradation of our food.

Two questions come to mind with these facts: if Americans didn't have refined and chemically tainted foods 200 years ago, then why were they dying so young? And if we are eating poorly today, why has our life expectancy rate increased? The answers have many facets.

Our bodies run on real food, and man developed over time to what we are today by eating real food. Back through time, without thinking, man reached out and consumed anything and everything that instinctively would satiate hunger, and generate survival. It was, in essence, survival of the fittest because there must have been mistakes made in choosing those bushes or berries that poisoned. And here we are, still trying to figure it out, and eat what we are meant to eat, and along the way trying to develop into super beings with improved longevity.

In examining the human diet of the past two centuries, some very interesting facts arise that the public rarely hears about. We may think that because foods could have been grown easily and organically, they must have been prevalent in the daily diet, but think again.

Thomas Tyron, an author during the 17th century, was a "healthy eating" advocate, trying to be a nutritionist of sorts for those times. He advocated vegetables, and began to condemn the slaughter of animals, but then backed off feeling too radical. In various writings he tried to teach how to cook cleaner, and prevent diseases. But when you don't have a national media system, the words go out to a select few, and finally fall on deaf ears.

Authors of the past centuries reveal eating habits of America and other countries. In the 1800s, French writer Constantin Francois de Volney was very descriptive in his account of visiting America, and observing the American eating habits. He wrote, "I will venture to say that if a prize were proposed for the scheme of a regimen most calculated to injure the stomach, the teeth, and the health in general, no better could be invented than that of the Americans." Every American meal was described as swimming in butter, hog's lard or fat, including the desserts.

European visitors to America during the early 1800s told of the state of the average American's health, reporting that they were a weak and tired people having crooked jaws, teeth missing, a grey pallor, a lazy gate, and overall health was dilapidated.

Salted meats were thought to be the most healthful food, salt pork being the most popular, and were served almost at every meal, depending on your wealth. Salt, at the time, was the major form of preservative. Peasants relied on breads and grains at breakfast, but during those times there was no refining of grains, and therefore the breads were more nutritious than the prestigious refined grains that the rich were paying to eat, and healthier than what we eat today.

Meats were considered a sign of prominence; the more aristocratic and wealthy you were, the more fresh meats were availed in each and every meal, along with an abundance of cheeses, nuts and sweets. The meats, however, were difficult to keep fresh, and often contained bacteria that, unbeknownst to the average person at the time, would cause various digestive problems, and even death. People, in fact, were equating most of these health problems to raw fruits and vegetables rather than the contaminated meats.

During the 1700s, raw fruit was thought to bring on indigestion or even the plague, therefore making it a common practice to boil all fruit. Rarely were they eaten raw; boiling fruits and vegetables, especially with salted pork, was the common mode of preparation, but were regarded as unnecessary, perhaps harmful. Vegetables such as cucumbers were thought to be 'noxious'. In Rousseau's writings during the 1700s, the word vegetable referred to milk, pastry and fruit.

Reverend Sylvester Graham, a Presbyterian minister during the 1800s, was a very vocal dietary reform advocate of whole wheat bread, as refining started to enter into the American diet. His book, *Treatise On Bread, and Bread Making*, told of the toll that refined flours had on the human body, warning that it caused diseases. He even told of the unwholesomeness of bread additives used at that time such as alum and chlorine. He preached that vegetables could cure alcoholism, and that meats caused sexual urges. He was threatened by butchers and bakers, and soon ridiculed by the public because of his rants.

What's interesting about Graham is that he invented the graham cracker for a more wholesome form of grains, and today it has turned into a food that is totally opposite of how his cracker was made, and of what he preached.

In 1900, the predominant causes of death were *(in this order)*:
1. Pneumonia
2. Influenza
3. Tuberculosis (1 in 7 died)
4. Gastrointestinal problems
5. Heart disease

Dental caries (infection) was a major cause of death between 1600-1800. By 1900, America was known to have the highest rates of tooth and gum disease anywhere in the world. Researchers noted that the teeth of the Native Americans confined to reservations were unstained and undamaged, and yet the average Caucasian had deteriorating teeth.

The cause of the rising amount of disease was attributed to the highly refined sugar and grains that Americans were suddenly eating, put together with low oral hygiene and improper dental maintenance and cleaning. Tooth decay had risen 35 times the amount of prehistoric Britain. Bacterial infection coming from the teeth was deduced to be tied to systemic diseases throughout the body, which included pneumonia.

Before the 20th century there were feeble means of keeping warm enough throughout the winters. It's currently expressed that cold weather does not cause colds and flu, however, studies point out that during cold weather cytokines become elevated causing inflammation in the airways that may create a susceptibility to pathogens that then affect the immune system. Infectious diseases can also be attributed to the lack of sunlight and its vitamin D during the winter months, as well as more people being in closed places susceptible to contamination from others. The industrial age brought more people living together with inadequate waste disposal and poor drinking water purification systems. Immune systems declined from poor, unclean living conditions and sanitation. Pneumonia, influenza and tuberculosis are all related to a deficient immune system.

Gastrointestinal problems abounded by the inferior food preservation and preparation techniques, with no awareness of contamination problems causing infection. A possible lack of fiber and enzymes could have played a part in intestinal distress.

Heart disease, contrary to the present, was commonly instigated by bacterial/infectious diseases and overuse of the common preservatives of alum, chlorine and salt; these were rubbed generously over most foods to help keep them from spoiling, and their abundant use added to heart disease and other ailments. Smoking was beginning to take on popularity in our society at the turn of the 20th century.

The proliferation of refined flours and sugar came in the 1800s. White sugar was a precious commodity as early as 500 A.D., but it was hard to come by, and very expensive. The wealthy during the 1500s were believed to have indulged greatly in it. From 1800 to 1900 came the huge turning point in refined sugar consumption for the masses.

Historical sugar consumption average per person:

   1700s - 4 pounds per year

   1800s - 18 pounds per year

   1900 - 90 pounds per year

Today, 2012, the average American consumes three pounds of sugar each week, or about **156 pounds** per year. This is not completely deliberate consumption of sugar, because a large part of the 156 pounds is hidden sugar in all the foods we either buy at the supermarket or eat at restaurants that we're not aware of.

In summation, these are major contributing factors to the low life expectancy before 1900:

1. Living conditions / sanitation
2. Lack of understanding importance of fruits/vegetables over meats
3. Rise of sugar consumption
4. Food preservation, preparation, contamination
5. Lack of injurious wound/infection care
6. Lack of drug treatments for survival
7. Initial rise of popularity with tobacco

Because of the lack of knowledge concerning foods and living conditions, societal health overall suffered. The increase of intelligence and discovery of sanitation, infection treatments, and development of drugs has brought about a longer life expectancy. Yet recently, this century, we are concerned with the degradation of our foods...refined flours and sugars, trans fats, hydrogenated oils, chemical preservatives, hormone injected meats, genetically modified foods, pesticides, lack of enzymes in cooked foods, and much more. This lack of awareness in food degradation has continued to stifle our life expectancy, not to mention our quality of life.

In 2000, the predominant causes of death were *(in this order)*:

1. Heart Disease
2. Cancer
3. Stroke
4. Accidents
5. Lung disease
6. Diabetes

(Cancer has tripled since 1900; heart disease is the number one cause of death since 1921.)

Instead of the immune system attacked by outside elements clearly being the culprit in the past, we now show more internal disruptions going on, all shown above, except for accidents. Smoking has contributed highly to our demise, but we have to look at what other toxins and altered substances go into our bodies daily that are creating havoc.

In summation, the major contributing factors to the influx of disease in and after the year 2000 are:

1. Smoking
2. Toxins/environmental/pharmaceutical chemicals
3. Processed foods/additives

With our ever-developing intelligence, we've eliminated the negative elements that affected us in the prior century, but we have clearly brought about these manufactured elements that can be linked to our demise.

We self inflict tobacco; manufacturers subject us to their toxins in farming, drugs, and everyday cleaning products, etc., which all find their way back into our water and ground supplies. And the food manufacturers subject us to, and leave us very little option than, ingesting substances that create imbalances, inflammation, and free radicals within our bodies causing disease: the degradation of the original foods, the chemicals used in processing, and chemicals/toxins that are part of the additives put into foods.

All causes of death for 2000 listed above are on the most part avoidable, if we all were to work together: the individual, the food growers, food manufacturers, and restaurants.

Keep in mind, our nation's obesity problem did not explode until the latter part of the 20th century. In 1980, childhood obesity was 7%, and in 2010 it rose to 18%, strongly correlating with an influx of refined foods, such as processed sugars, grains and oils.

*"Those who think they have no time for healthy eating,
will sooner or later have to find time for illness"*

~ Edward Stanley

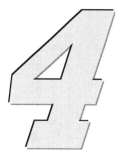

Chapter 4

What's Wrong With This Picture?

Take a serious look at what you have for breakfast, lunch and dinner. What's in your cereal besides grains? Is your juice fresh from the fruit? Is your turkey fresh from the turkey, or is it processed?

The meats have additives to keep them fresh. The animals the meat comes from have been injected with hormones and chemicals to make them produce more meat, and keep them from contracting diseases. The cereals are overly processed and have processed sugars added. Pesticides find their way into our fruits and vegetables. Canned and bottled foods have devalued vitamins and minerals, and enzymes are destroyed. Even our drinking water is suspect; toxic fluoride and chlorine are common additives.

We all have to do the best we can with the choices given to us by our food suppliers. The main food suppliers in our lives at the present time are the supermarkets and fast-food restaurants. What is offered to us in our supermarket food supply has been produced on the most part in a way to increase profits for the food manufacturers and distributors; not to increase our state of health. They want longer shelf life, more attractive, unflawed fruit, and the cheapest ways to process and package.

When you add everything up, we would have to stop eating everything sold in a supermarket, and grow our own food, and raise our own chickens, in order to be assured of avoiding the harmful additives that we unknowingly ingest daily. Take a look at high fructose corn syrup, now the number one sugar additive being used today in the U.S. It's not only the most harmful form of sugar created by man for man, it has crept into our food without warning or approval.

Most of the commercial cooking oils are highly processed and molecularly altered; most sugars and sweeteners, including agave, the latest fad sugar, are highly processed, molecularly altered, or contain chemicals; most "fresh" fruit is cold-stored for months before reaching the supermarket; pigs, cows and cattle are injected with hormones and antibiotics that can disrupt the human internal system…hormone imbalance and resistance to antibiotics. Pesticides seep into vegetables through the soil and water system. Going organic is the best choice, but at the moment, can we trust every label marked organic?

It is very difficult to get the big picture on how our food sources have evolved over time to the state they are in today. It's unfortunate that over the years Americans have had no input to the approval process of food manufacturing. With our eager acceptance of convenience we have given free reign to the food manufacturers for what goes into the foods we eat, and this has been going on for decades.

It is not feasible to force people into an abrupt change to totally raw foods and foreign tastes, but to help everyone see the light and make subtle changes over time that could help turn health around.

Consciously we can take charge of our lives; it's the current unconscious motions we go through in choosing our daily diet that is troublesome. We grab what's predominantly available rather than putting any thought into what's in it, where it comes from, and what are the pros and cons.

Here is a look at the evolution of our food supply over the last 200 years or so, which has affected our nation's health. Think about how your health may improve if you were to change certain foods on this list on a daily basis. Over time, your body would definitely benefit by not having to combat the ill effects of deficient, toxic and nutritionally imbalanced foods.

Top Twelve areas of our food that have had uncontested, detrimental changes in our diet over the last 200 years:

1. Canned Foods

2. Baby Formula

3. Refined Flour

4. Sugared Drinks

5. Hydrogenated Oils

6. Homogenized/Pasteurized Milk

7. Use of Plastic Food and Drink Packaging

8. Grain Fed/Hormone and Antibiotic Injected Meats

9. Food Hybridization/Manipulation

10. High Fructose Corn Syrup

11. Farmed Fish

12. Genetically Modified Foods (Organisms) (GMO)

1. 1812 - Canned Foods

In 1812 the idea of "tinned" foods came to the United States from France. Napoleon instigated the invention by wanting to find a way to preserve the foods being sent to his troops in war. The French were the first to invent a preservation method with bottles, but the first canning facility was established in the United States in 1812.

While canning fruits and vegetables is a very viable way of getting them to areas where it is difficult to obtain such foods, or providing certain people or populations with foods that will keep them alive, it is never the best option in trying to stay healthy. The heating process in canning foods kills a high percentage of vitamins and minerals, and then again as the consumer heats the contents before eating, more precious nutrients are lost; the highly beneficial enzymes are totally eliminated through the heat process. Enzymes are a vital part of the human diet. To go through life without consuming these naturally contributive digestive aids found in raw fruits and vegetables taxes the pancreas, and can eventually lower life expectancy.

Also, manufacturers choose to add an unnecessary amount of salt and sugar to certain canned foods, not only for preservative measures but also to just make the foods more tasteful (more marketable) to eat.

It has been recently reported that the toxic chemical BPA has been found in canned foods at health-threatening amounts. It has long been an ingredient in the epoxy resin lining of the cans over the last few decades but the figures reported were not alarming. Now new findings are showing harmful amounts for the consumer. The more canned foods eaten, the more BPA enters the body. BPA is already (and has been for several years) under scrutiny for consumer exposure in plastic bottles – most importantly baby bottles - but the fight to eliminate it from our food and water containers has been and will still be an arduous task. The canning process itself also results in producing chemical reactions in the food that contribute to inflammation in the body.

There are certain companies that now use BPA-free cans, and more will follow. It's unfortunate they don't advertise this important feature, but you can do your homework online if you'd like to search them out. If all manufacturers were to begin using non-BPA cans, this toxic exposure would cease; it has been proposed to do just that in the near future.

This being said, the use of canned foods should still be limited by consumers. Canned fruits and vegetables should always be avoided, and instead use fresh or frozen. Such foods as BPA-free canned legumes (pinto beans, etc.), salmon and meats, which need to be cooked well anyway, can be a convenient source, as long as they are without additives.

2. 1869 - Baby Formula

Around 1869 the first commercial baby formula was marketed out of a growing concern for infants getting inadequate nourishment. One of the first formulas included potassium bicarbonate, wheat flour and malt flour that was added to warmed cow's milk. Another formula, called Farine Lactee, was sugar, and flour or cornmeal, mixed with either milk or water. Quite basic, but at least it was an attempt to save the lives of newborns who were not able to consume breast milk for some reason. It was soon discovered that deaths among formula-fed babies far outnumbered the breast-fed babies.

Over many decades, after an acceptable formula came on the market, doctors began promoting the use of formula instead of breastfeeding, and along with successful marketing, baby formula sales peeked in the 1970s, feeding 75% of newborns.

There are hundreds of ingredients within natural breast milk, and still today the entire unique qualities and ingredients of breast milk cannot be duplicated in man-made baby formula. Babies fed formula exclusively miss out on the number one defense ingredient of breast milk, colostrum. This natural occurring substance is inherent in all nursing mammals, and contains enhanced immune and growth factors naturally made to naturally protect against disease, immune deficiency problems and toxins, including those found in vaccines. During the first 72 hours as the baby suckles its mother, this substance, not basic milk, comes from the breast to the baby, filled with all the special nutrients a virgin intestinal tract needs to become prepared for the foods from the earth and the damaging processed foods soon to be ingested. Without the natural ingredients of breast milk, damage to the system could possibly affect a person's state of health throughout life. For this reason baby formula definitely should be scrutinized as a contributor to immunity diseases, gastrointestinal disorders, allergies, Type 1 diabetes, autism, and more.

Damage may in fact come mainly from the ingredients in infant formula - the presence of unnatural cow's milk (a known allergen), processed oils, refined sugars, synthetic vitamins and minerals. All ingredients are pasteurized, killing needed good probiotic bacteria. And to top it off, the entire ingredients are prepared under manufacturing plant conditions. They may be overseen by The Food Safety and Inspection Service (FSIS), but still cannot be 100% void of any contaminations with such elaborate processing. Without breast milk, the substitute of formula reaches the child's intestinal tract before it has a chance to become nutritionally guarded against those very foreign substances. One such substance that is highly suspect is one of two cow proteins. These are named as possible contributors to Type 1 diabetes and asthma.

3. 1880s – Refined Flour

Grains, at the beginning of their consumption, were always eaten whole without major processing; who's to say they didn't just pluck it out of the ground and eat. Grinding was the first grain process for mass consumption. A lighter, less coarse flour came to be in Roman times, as the sifting process was discovered – producing white refined flour by removing the course, protective outer shell (bran) and the embryo (germ). Refined flour gave a smooth desirable texture that people began to prefer, but only the wealthy could afford such breads since it was more expensive to produce. The lower class could only afford the common unrefined bread – which contained all the nutrients. Now it is just the opposite; the non-nutritious refined breads are affordable to those of lesser means.

In the 1920s, deficiency diseases began to occur such as pellagra, caused by the lack of niacin, and beriberi, caused by the deficiency of thiamine (B1), major nutrients inherent to whole grain. In 1941 it was mandated by the government that flour be fortified with various vitamins in order to prevent these diseases. Now, we no longer are in danger of contracting pellagra since they add the missing vitamins, but these added vitamins are of lesser quality than what is naturally inherent. Our refined flours today are still deficient in other nutrients and fiber associated with the bran and the germ.

Refined flours are the cause of increased blood pressure, diabetes and heart disease by the fact that there is limited fiber to slow the process of digestion; the glucose from grains rapidly assimilates into the bloodstream causing the inflammation that triggers the subsequent diseases like diabetes and arterial damage. In addition to the missing nutrients, modern refined flour products are exposed to nearly 70 chemicals used for the processing of commercial flour: bleaching agents, improving agents, raising agents, enzyme active preparation, yeast stimulators, preservatives, emulsifiers, stabilizers, coloring agents, acids, just to name a few.

4. 1880s - Refined Sugar/Sugared Drinks

Ireland introduced "Ginger Ale" in the 1850s, as the first commercial sugared drink. In America the ice cream sodas became popular; then in 1876, Root Beer was mass-produced, spawning the start of the commercial drinks of Dr. Pepper and Coca-Cola. And so the daily consumption of "sugar water" began. The average American child consumes about 10 tablespoons of sugar each day, and the average American adult consumes about 7. The American Heart Association recommends no more than 3 tablespoons a day. There are over 3 tablespoons of sugar in one can of Coca-Cola. Besides the soft drink fix, we consume sugar when we eat catsup, mayonnaise, yogurt, salad dressing, breads, desserts, stewed tomatoes, breakfast cereals, and the list goes on and on. The sugars are never really required in the making of most of these foods; they are merely added to help their products sell. Consumers crave and want that sweet taste, and that's what sells. The three main sources of sugar are sugar cane, beets, and corn that are converted into sweeteners for the various food products. Sugared drinks have become a staple in the American diet. It's never unusual to see children everywhere carrying bottles of sugar water with them wherever they go. Whether eating meals out at a restaurant or at home, a sugared drink is now most likely consumed by the average American family with every meal. Sugar is running through the arteries of most Americans most of their waking hours. It has become the number one food quantity (other than meat) to be consumed by Americans daily. In a study, it was found that animals eating sugar and water died before those that just drank water.

5. 1900 - Pasteurized Milk / Homogenized Milk

Pasteurization of milk became popular first in the late 1800s in Europe, and during the early 1900s in the United States. In 1938, milk products were the cause of 25% of the food and waterborne illnesses and/or deaths; they now account for 1%. Raw, natural milk was a mainstay in the human diet for thousands of years, but as populations grew, the production and dissemination of milk products grew without regard to any health risks that may be connected to housing animals, packaging milk products, and the hauling and storage. Because it's a "live food", microorganisms are a threat, as is the sanitation regarding the animals and the hands of the milkers and packagers involved. The contamination of the milk soon got out of hand, and it was much easier to sterilize the milk rather than sterilizing the surroundings, the cows and hands of the workers. Chicago, in 1908, was the first city to make pasteurization mandatory for milk sold within the city.

One faction at the time advocated for *certified raw milk*, meaning the process and facilities would raise the standards of the dairy industry and be closely monitored in order to distribute a safe product. The other faction advocated for pasteurization, stating the raw milk process would be costly. It came down to a matter of economics – pasteurization would save money, and be an easier and quick fix.

Pasteurization and homogenization of milk has turned it into a processed food. It contributes to inflammation of the arteries, and, as noted above, milk is implicated in various adverse health conditions.

6. 1911 - Hydrogenated Oils

A French chemist first developed the hydrogenation process for oils in the 1890s in order for processed, packaged foods to have a longer shelf life. Crisco by Procter & Gamble was the first food product to contain hydrogenated oils, or "trans fat", in the U.S, commercialized in 1911. By 1930, the use of hydrogenated oils was widespread. The chemical structure of heated, hydrogenated oils are so altered that the oils come close to resembling a plastic in molecular structure. The most highly processed oils are corn, cotton, soy and canola. It has been found that these highly processed oils can thicken the blood, make the heart work harder, contribute to inflammation and high blood pressure. It's another food lacking enzymes, which causes the body to utilize its own enzymes in the digestion process of such foods, also causing the liver to work harder. It affects the permeability of cell walls, causing inflammation in the arteries, and can lead to heart disease, tumors, cancer and other diseases. These hydrogenated oils are commonly found in most boxed foods, commercial bakery goods, margarines, and often hidden in restaurant foods. It is not only the worst oil to be used by man (and created by man), but the FDA actually allows a company to have .5% of a hydrogenated oil added to products without the manufacturer having to say that their product contains "trans fat", now deemed by the FDA to be anti-nutritious.

7. 1930 - Food Hybridization/Manipulation

Hybridization, the art of creating the 'perfect' crop, can produce grains that are resistant to bugs and diseases, or alter how or where it grows. The balance of minerals and vitamins in these crops can be changed; some become unnaturally high in sugar, and suspect in contributing to candida, a fungas that can reside in our bodies. It creates an unnatural food source that our bodies may not recognize.

These are foods that have been altered in some way in order to make food taste better, to make food more resistant to herbicides, to make food stay fresh longer, and/or to merely make them void of seeds, as with watermelons.

A *new* wheat was created in the sixties that was named 'dwarf wheat'. It was developed to answer the need for a higher yield of wheat especially in under-developed countries. This new species does not need to grow as high, and will grow in a shorter period of time. Its use caught on in America. This new wheat has more gluten, more starch, and creates more inflammation and higher blood sugar than regular wheat. Our fast foods are full of it.

Manipulation of foods can go something like this: Tomatoes on the market today are very often picked when they are green, gassed with ethylene to develop their red color, and refrigerated for as long as it takes to be distributed. Many fruits such as apples are treated with preservatives as soon as they are picked, and waxed with shellac or carnuba wax. They are then refrigerated at 32 degrees at a reduced level of oxygen, and possibly stored for three months before heading to the supermarkets.

8. 1949 – Use of Plastic Food and Drink Packaging

Our use of plastics surrounding our food products has become excessively prolific since its start in 1949. The food packaging companies were first with its use, and then products for the kitchen were developed around 1953, such as plastic wrap and containers. In 1970 came the first plastic soft drink bottles, replacing glass. These plastic items are now filling our landfills, but the immediate threat from them is the toxic contaminants that exude into our foods and drinks. Plastics used in food wrap, containers and bottles have shown to release various toxic chemicals such as dioxins, DEHA, and BPA, especially when exposed to high temperatures and the microwave. Never heat plastic containers and reuse them, and never leave a plastic bottle in the hot sun or a hot car.

Concerning plastics in the food industry, there is controversy between the FDA and the health communities; the FDA maintains these plastics are not a major threat, and so they allow its use to continue; and the health community believes that the more plastic humans are exposed to, the more threat to their health. In thinking about how much plastic we, and our foods, are exposed to, it's best to try to keep it to a minimum, and away from foods as much as possible.

9. 1950 - Grain Fed, Hormone and Antibiotic Injected Meats

Prior to World War II, cattle grazed on green wholesome grass throughout the country to fatten up for market. After World War II, U.S. farmers began to produce more grain than they could sell, and so it was fed to cows. Not only does it quickly fatten up the cattle and poultry, and produce more milk, it fattens humans as well as we drink the milk and eat the beef. Also, the grain-induced meats are highly inflammatory to our bodies, unbalancing our diet with omega 6 oils, the oils that we have an over abundance in our daily diet already. The grass-fed meats that we should be eating induce the opposite; grass-fed steers and cows produce beef and milk with the highly needed omega 3 oils.

Growth hormone supplementation first took place in 1947 at Purdue University as a study. The procedure was approved by the FDA in 1954, and was rapidly adopted in the meat industry. One form of growth hormone was found in the 1970s to cause cancer, and was banned. It is a standard for most American cattle to be given steroids/hormones in order to produce *leaner* meat and promote faster growth. One controversy is that hormones given to the cattle pass on to humans, and the over-ingestion and stimulation of these hormones can cause unhealthy disturbances within the human body.

The USDA does not allow the use of hormones in hogs and poultry, and therefore these meats do not need to advertise the term "no hormones added", but some companies do, just to catch attention.

About 80% of the antibiotics sold in the United States are used for meat and poultry production to prevent diseases caused by crowding and unsanitary conditions at these farms. Chickens producing free-range and organic eggs cannot, by law, be injected with antibiotics. Antibiotics given to animals are passed on to the consumer, and can contribute to drug resistance, making common antibiotics given for human illness ineffective. A buildup of these inherited antibiotics in food add toxins to the body that contribute to disease.

10. 1970 - High Fructose Corn Syrup

The public now is becoming more aware of the sugar additive called high fructose corn syrup, and manufacturers have begun to eliminate the use of this detrimental substance yet it is still pervasive. HFCS came to be in 1957, and introduced in our diet on an industrial scale in the 1970s. In order to make soft drinks cheaper to produce, the American manufacturers began around 1984 to use HFCS, made from corn, a cheaper source of sugar, instead of refined sugar cane. (Most foreign soft drink manufacturers still use sugar, including Coca-Cola overseas' production.) HFCS is actually a refined product made from an already refined product...cornstarch. Because of its extreme refinement, HFCS health issues include a higher risk of diabetes, higher risk of weight gain or obesity, hypertension, and liver damage. And, rarely noted, it contains a high level of mercury from the processing method, among other chemicals, resulting in brain and nerve damage. HFCS is found in various salad dressings, sodas, fruit juices, bakery goods and commercial breads.

11. 1970 - Farmed Fish

The fish farm industry began in Canada in the 70s, grew in the U.S. around 1990, and now accounts for 80% of the fish consumed in the U.S. Because there are high numbers of fish housed in contained areas, they are susceptible to disease and thus administered antibiotics to keep them alive. The amount of antibiotics given to fish exceeds the amount the livestock industry uses (in relation to animal weight), and these antibiotics are passed on to the consumer. The carcinogenic toxins found in farmed fish include PCBs and dioxin. In farmed salmon, they have found ten times more toxins than wild salmon.

Unfortunately, farmed salmon are not fed the usual wild salmon diet of zooplankton, small invertebrates, herring, or krill. They are fed corn, soy and other grains, causing extreme inflammation to the end consumer, us. Since the farmed salmon do not eat their usual foods, they do not become the beautiful pink color they should be, and then must be treated with chemicals to make their flesh turn to pink.

12. 1994 - Genetically Modified Foods (Organisms) (GMO)

GMO foods are those altered by high-tech complex laboratory methods that can include gene splitting. They can cross genetic material from different species, whereby hybridization involves same-specie manipulation. The consumer unfortunately is mostly unaware of these products because they do not have to be labeled as such.

In 1994 Monsanto introduced the genetically engineered growth hormone recombinant bovine somatotropin (rBST), or bovine growth hormone (BGH)), to boost dairy output. It's interesting to note that tobacco was one of the first crops to be genetically engineered, at the same time as the first GM tomato.

GMO foods can cause allergies and inflammation at the least. The possible highly damaging effects are speculated to be DNA integration and alteration, antibiotic resistance, cancer and more. In France, a two-year study, published in *Food and Chemical Toxicology*, claims that tumors were two to three times more prevalent in mice that were fed a diet that consisted of 11 percent GM corn. The USDA Economic Research Service reported that possibly 90 percent of corn chips sold have been genetically modified in some way.

Unfortunately GMO foods are sneaking into our food supply more and more recently, undetected. They are yet to be mandatorily labeled as such, or controlled by the FDA.

"The doctor of the future will no longer treat the human frame with drugs, but rather will cure and prevent disease with nutrition"

~ *Thomas Edison*

Chapter 5

Re-thinking Breakfast

It's not surprising that many people do not eat a proper breakfast, and there are far too many who don't even eat breakfast at all; both are unhealthful. Our bodies need fuel in the morning to get started. After sleeping for many hours, our bodies naturally use up energy, fluids, nutrients, just in recalibrating – body tissue is renewed, human growth hormone is produced, and a natural cancer fighter (TNF) inherent to our immune system is spawned ten times more than during waking hours.

It's a good idea to have fuel enter the body slowly in the morning, without heavy digestion going on, without putting much pressure on the system. Whole fruit is a perfect type of food and fuel to start the day. So many feel the need for a cup of coffee in the morning, but the glucose, our main energy source, gained from a bowl of fruit will energize the brain cells.

The brain utilizes a large amount of our glucose consumption, and glucose is the only form of sugar the brain will utilize, and too much fructose will slow brain function. The brain does not store glucose, so once it travels to the brain, we are awake and ready to go. The cup of coffee won't hurt most; it's what you put into it, and how much caffeine you consume. Whole fruit can be a great substitute for many.

The typical American breakfast has evolved into an overload of refined sugar or fast-acting glucose-producing refined products, and most often without proper protein. Protein can help slow down the release of sugar into the bloodstream.

Typical breakfast choices are usually:

- Cereal - *glucose*
- Bagel, Toast or Muffin - *glucose*
- Coffee
- Smoothie – *fructose/glucose*
- Fruit Juice – *fructose/glucose*
- Milk/Yogurt – *lactose/glucose*

Cereal – Most breakfast cereal products contain added sugar substances; but even if they don't, the grains they are made from naturally convert to glucose/sugar in the body. And because most grains used are without bran and germ, ground to a flour and pressed into shapes, they turn to sugar much quicker, causing inflammation.

Bagels, Toast, Muffins – Again, usually refined flour, these grains turn into glucose/sugar in the body.

Coffee – Most likely the average coffee drinker is not drinking coffee plain, but with added refined sugar substances and the non-dairy creamer made from unhealthful ingredients such as corn syrup and hydrogenated oils.

Smoothies – If these are made at a smoothie outlet, then there is a possibility there is some sort of refined sugar included, or a commercial fruit juice has been included that has no fiber and no enzymes. Many homemade smoothies most often contain more sugar than protein. Processed fruit takes less time to enter the blood stream and turns into glucose quickly, inflaming the arteries on the way while it raises the blood sugar level. This creates inflammation.

Fruit Juices – Any fruit juice speeds through to the blood stream and rapidly inflames the arteries on the way. The juice without the fiber travels faster and causes more havoc; the juice with fiber at least slows it down and helps control inflammation and blood pressure somewhat. Commercial canned, bottled, packaged fruit juices are void of enzymes and have lost a large percent of the natural vitamins and minerals, not to mention the fiber.

Milk/Yogurt – Milk is often a daily beverage staple and/or used for cereal in the morning. It's not commonly known, but milk, as well as yogurt, also contains its own natural sugar, lactose.

Glucose is obviously the attraction to these foods in the morning as glucose can get the adrenalin running, and unfortunately a high percentage of breakfast meals contain a high amount of fructose these days.

Protein has been forgotten in the American homemade breakfast, mainly because of the lack of time people have to fix a meal before going to work. One of the best proteins has been eliminated with most people because of a bad reputation for having a load of cholesterol. This fear of eggs has recently been discredited, as it's explained in Chapter 6.

Where has the protein and fiber gone in our breakfast? Protein tends to be consumed more often when people eat breakfast out.

We all can recognize this following breakfast as one typically eaten at restaurants:

- Pancakes or waffles, with refined sugar-based syrup, whipped cream
- Bacon or sausage
- Eggs
- Juice
- Toast w/jam

An overload of sugars once again, and an abundance of saturated animal fats become the main protein. For those who make the typical quick breakfast at home every day before going to work, eating breakfast at a restaurant is welcomed as a treat or reward for the hard work or long hours you've put in all week, and therefore people indulge themselves with a meal that is more of a dessert, and a time of accepting their rare intake of eggs (since they still believe eggs are bad for them) as a reward for going without for so long. But eggs do not have to be avoided anytime. They make the best protein source we have – low saturated fat, and easily digestible.

There are several good protein options for breakfast; here is a list of them, and how many grams of protein in each:

1 Egg	6 grams
Smoked Salmon	5-10 grams
1/2 cup Cashews	10 grams
2 TBLS Cashew Butter	6 grams
1/2 cup Almonds	12 grams
2 TBLS Almond Butter	4 grams
1/2 cup Macadamia Nuts	5 grams
1/2 cup cooked Beans	8 grams
1 cup Oatmeal	6 grams
Chicken Thigh, 1/4 Breast	7-10 grams
1 cup Quinoa	8 grams
Homemade Veggie Burger	5-10 grams

Don't be afraid to eat lunch for breakfast...

There is no reason we can't break away from the traditional breakfasts of cereal and toast or yogurt, and instead have a turkey sandwich or a bowl of soup. Have that leftover piece of chicken with some sprouted grain toast.

There are healthful cereal choices, and they include oatmeal, amaranth, quinoa and puffed brown rice or millet. These are true whole grain cereals; they are not ground into flour, and do not come with added sugar. There is no significant nutritional difference between steel-cut and regular oats. Both forms retain all their original parts. These grains are also great for an afternoon or late-night snack.

Basically, cereal means ground to a flour. For typical cereal, flour is then shaped into flakes or circles or waffles or honeycombs, to become whatever the manufacturer wants to market to children and adults. It's the grinding to a powdery flour, as well as the refining of the grain (removing the bran and germ), that gets our arteries into trouble.

Keep in mind that before a hearty breakfast everyone should follow an added health ritual to go along with your body waking up in the morning. This ritual could become commonplace with everyone's morning routine:

1. Upon rising, always drink a full glass of water to cleanse the system.

2. Eat whole fruit before anything else to get the intestinal tract ready to accept the heavier foods; fruits are fiber-filled, natural sugar, and digest easier than most other foods. Another healthful practice is to eat fruit separate from grains and proteins since a fermentation process begins when they combine, and for many people with intestinal problems, this would exacerbate whatever condition is present. Wait at least 20-30 minutes to have your breakfast protein or grains.

3. Never drink fruit juice.

4. Always include a protein for breakfast, to slow the absorption of glucose. Many good protein meals can be fixed the night before.

Alternatives to the typical breakfast, can be leftovers or premade dishes:

- Chicken Vegetable Soup
- Smoked Salmon w/capers or pesto sauce on sprouted toast
- Mediterranean Salad
- Chicken Salad
- Tuna Salad
- Leftover meats from day before with vegetables (celery stalk, radishes, tomatoes, etc.)
- Blended Vegetable Drink w/ turkey slices
- Healthy Chocolate/Banana Shake w/raw egg
- Sweet Potato, Peppers and Onions
- Quinoa with golden raisins, nuts, apples and cinnamon
- Mashed black, red or pinto beans w/cilantro, onions in a 100% brown rice tortilla
- Turkey breakfast sausage w/tomato wedges and onions

Put on your thinking cap for some unique breakfast choices.

"Healthy is merely the slowest rate at which one can die"

~ Author Unknown

Chapter 6

Concerns for Moving in the Right Direction

- Top Concerns for Health Maintenance
- Cooking Tips to Improve Your Heath
- Healthful Kitchen Habits
- Recipe Replacements
- Supermarket Purchasing Tips
- Commercial Everyday Foods Containing Sugar (or sugar substitutes) that can easily be avoided
- Worst Foods to Purchase
- Easy Between-Meals Snacks
- Top Restaurant Foods Not to Trust
- Changes Needed by Food Providers
- Most Underrated Foods
- Most Overrated Foods
- Top Anti-Inflammatory Foods
- Top Antioxidant Foods
- Top Supplements to Take Daily
- Top Anti-Inflammatory/Antioxidant Supplements

Top Concerns for Health Maintenance

- Acid/Alkaline balance
- Inflammation/Inflammatory foods
- Blood Sugar/Insulin
- Enzymes
- Immune System
- Hormones

Most of the public is unaware of the true explanation of cholesterol's role in the body, which is explained on page 92 (Eggs), showing why it is not a top concern. There is a definite relationship between cholesterol, inflammation and the acid/alkaline balance. By concentrating on alkaline and anti-inflammatory foods, concern with cholesterol will diminish.

1. Alkaline/Acid Balance

There are foods that create alkaline within the body (mostly fruits and vegetables) and foods that create an acidic reaction. For a balanced body, and to stave off disease, at least a 60/40 ratio of alkaline and acid pH foods should be consumed. This balance is mainly affected by the foods we eat. We do need a small amount of acidic foods in order to keep alive, but because our Western diet is so inundated with "fast foods" that include refined grains (acid), sugars (acid), trans fats/hydrogenated oils (acid), high fructose corn syrup (acid), and high meat intake (acid), especially cattle that are fed on grains (more acid), then we are absorbing too much acidic components that will eventually disease our system. The therapeutic ratio of alkaline/acid should be 80/20 in dealing with threatening, debilitating disease; 70/30 is optimum for maintenance; 60/40 ratio is healthful. (*See Chapter 9, Food Health Factor Reference Chart.*)

Remember, the more a food is processed or refined, the more acidic it will be to the body.

2. Inflammation/Inflammatory foods

There are certain types of foods that create an inflammatory response in the body, and there are foods that are known anti-inflammatory, meaning they can counteract the effects of the inflammatory foods. Antioxidant-rich and anti-inflammatory foods go hand in hand. Inflammation has been determined as a major factor in artery/heart disease, bowel disease, high blood pressure, and many more types of health concerns. It is mostly the altered foods perceived as alien to our body that do harm to our arteries and intestinal walls thus creating an inflammation response. On the most part, these foods are inflammatory because our body sees them as foreign, unknown, unnatural substances that do not harmonize in our system. There are some natural, healthful foods, mostly fruits, that have been deemed as inflammatory (See Chapter 9, *Food Health Factor Reference Chart*) in the inflammation analysis mainly because of their high sugar or fructose content; however, most fruits contain strong anti-inflammatory components plus high fiber that negate the high sugar content claim of inflammation. High fructose consumption, especially the additive high fructose corn syrup, has been implicated in disease susceptibility, and it would be ardent to just consciously make a point to eat more vegetables than fruits to lower your overall intake of sugar.

Remember, the more a food is processed or refined, the more inflammatory it will be to the body.

3. Blood Sugar/Insulin

Eating too much refined foods, sugars and flours, will cause the liver and pancreas to malfunction, putting the body into a diabetic situation. Unfortunately, the word does not get out that Type 2 diabetes can be reversed and eliminated by diet and nutrition. The public is basically lulled into thinking that diabetes is something that will not go away, and must be treated by drugs forever. Some are not even being told it is a diet-related condition. Eating more fiber, more vegetables, and no refined foods will keep the body void of insulin resistance and diabetes. Most diabetics should eliminate all fruit until they get their issue controlled naturally. (Contact a certified nutritionist to help.) Far too many people are misdiagnosed, or not diagnosed early enough. It's the insulin level that needs to be checked, and not just the blood sugar level for determining true diabetes. The *insulin response test,* done while fasting, is the proper test to take to see if you are at risk. Too much insulin in the system is the road to diabetes. Insulin resistance develops, and shuts down the source. Lifestyle changes are necessary to lower insulin production. It's predicted that half of Americans will have diabetes by 2020 unless the proper information is given to the public in order to make the proper diet changes.

4. Enzymes

The foods we eat need to be broken down before the nutrients can be assimilated into our system. Enzymes are natural components found in all uncooked, unpackaged, unprocessed foods; from raw fruits, vegetables, and eggs to raw steak, enzymes are within each and every *live* food to help the body digest each particular food. When any *live* food is cooked, gone are the enzymes. Any canned, jarred, bottled food or liquid, including dairy products, has been depleted of enzymes through pasteurization. When a food lacking enzymes is introduced into the body, the stomach or pancreas are signaled that enzymes are lacking, and then the needed enzymes are sent over to the stomach with digestive juices to help in the digestion process. Even the simple act of chewing gum will send a signal to the pancreas that digestion needs to take place, and enzymes are needed. This is a false alarm, using up precious enzymes.

The enzymes produced by our own body come from a natural *back-up* system, but this supply can deplete if over-used throughout one's life, as with someone eating a constant diet of fried, boiled, and processed food. The pancreas and its enzyme store could stop working properly because of the major burden put upon it. The younger a person begins a diet of mostly cooked, packaged foods, the sooner that enzyme store may deplete.

The only alternative in this case is to either stop eating or lower your intake of cooked and altered foods, or supply the body with enzyme supplements every time cooked or processed food is eaten. There are enzymes for every type of food eaten, and there are quality, comprehensive digestive enzyme supplements that everyone would benefit by taking daily with meals to help with digestion of cooked foods. This is why it is so important to eat as many raw foods as possible. Raw honey and extra virgin olive and other oils prove to have very high amounts of natural enzymes.

Digestive enzymes are not the only type of enzymes we have; there are thousands of different types that work in magical ways to help our systems function properly. When supplemental enzymes are taken without food present, they go to work finding irregularities within the system to help correct. No one can get too many supplemental enzymes, especially when disease is present. Ask your nutritionist the best source for these.

There are foods, however, that are natural antagonists to our enzyme system; these include any food that has a naturally long shelf-life, and are: nuts, legumes, seeds, grains.

Every food has its inherent defenses against invaders, just as we have with our immune system. The nuts, legumes, seeds and grains have what are called *enzyme inhibitors*. These are present to keep these foods intact until they are presented with moisture. These foods have been *programmed* to wait out time in order to be bathed in water so it can germinate, and then release its nutrients. It's about propagation. Unfortunately for us, when we eat these foods raw or cooked before they were allowed to sprout, then we are ingesting those enzyme inhibitors that will thus neutralize some of our own enzymes within our system. They also bind with precious minerals such as calcium, magnesium, iron and zinc, blocking them from absorption by our bodies. Cooking will eliminate most of the inhibitors, but then that will destroy also all the enzymes as well that aid digestion. Raw peanuts and raw wheat germ have very large amounts of enzyme inhibitors.

By eating too many of these particular raw foods, we lose enzymes and nutrients. But there is one very good remedy for being able to eat these raw foods without the loss of enzymes and nutrients, and that is by soaking and sprouting.

Sprouting legumes, nuts and seeds can easily be done at home, and there are more and more sprouted foods coming onto the market for our convenience, from sprouted nuts to sprouted breads and cereal. This is the type of convenience food for our own good, and should become more and more popular.

5. Immune System

The immune system is our major defense from illness, yet it is not a specific organ like the kidney or liver. The immune system is comprised of several elements/components spread throughout the body, basic areas that include but not limited to the spleen, lymph nodes, and skin. The gut, or intestinal tract, is considered ground zero of our immune system, the thymus gland the king (at the base of the neck). If these two areas are deficient, then the body's main defenses are down, allowing foreign invaders to wreak havoc and cause illness. By how we treat our bodies, and by eating certain foods, we can either suppress our immune system or support it. The main supporters of the gut and thymus are:

- Probiotics
- Herbs
- Vegetables
- Antioxidants
- Exercise

Elevating the amount of probiotics that live naturally in the intestines (the bacterial defenders) will ward off the bad bacteria we acquire from toxins, bad foods, prescription drugs, etc.

Taking an antibiotic for infection will quickly kill the good bacteria (probiotics), and leave the body vulnerable. Antibiotics are far over-prescribed in our society today, and we need to think more about if and when we really need to take them. It has become common thinking that the antibiotic is the easiest and most reliable way to get well, when in fact in most cases, without a fever, sore throats, ear infections, the flu and the like will be cured by the body itself in time. Many people don't realize that antibiotics do not cure the flu or colds; they are for infection only. But whenever antibiotics are administered, a good probiotic needs to be taken as well, but not at the same time or those good bacteria will be destroyed with the bad. Take them two hours apart.

Free radicals (the foreign invaders produced by toxins, chemicals, altered food molecules) jeopardize the thymus, and antioxidants will fight them. Fresh herbs and vegetables hold the proper minerals, vitamins and micronutrients that protect and enhance our thymus as well as every cell in our body.

The more blood flow is increased throughout the body, primarily with exercise, the more waste products that affect the thymus and lymph nodes will be thrust from the system. Saunas are another means for pulling the toxins out of the body.

A deficient immune system will ultimately allow disease to form. One spectrum of disease is what is known as autoimmune disorders, which actually encompass a gamut of disease types; these are multiple sclerosis (MS), rheumatoid arthritis, Crohn's disease, lupus, Hashimoto's thyroiditis, Grave's, and psoriasis. Other smaller forms can go undetected, and cause various smaller problems within the body without you or your doctor realizing it is an autoimmune response. Unfortunately you could be misdiagnosed, and put on drugs that don't address the real problem. It's an area that the medical community is still trying to figure out.

As with MS, it's looked at as a 'disease' in itself, but there can be many factors. Autoimmunity develops when the immune system is so jeopardized that when a foreign invader begins to disrupt the system, the body will attack its own tissues rather than the invading predator. Hashimoto's is not a thyroid dysfunction, it is an inadequate, confused immune system attacking the thyroid.

Autoimmune disorders tend to develop from a *perfect storm* of circumstances, generally comprised of trauma/stress, food allergies and altered foods, toxins, and over-stimulation of prescription drugs. It does not seem to be caused by one thing. The system becomes so confused by different triggers transpiring at the same time, and begins to attack itself.

This form of immune imbalance seems to be becoming a major area of disease in our society lately, and could develop into numbers close to those of diabetes. We have become a society with over-prescribed drugs and foods containing anti-nutrients, both causing deficient immune systems; add the stress or trauma, and it's a formula for system failure.

6. Hormones

Hormones are very important components of the body as they are the catalyst for things to happen by sending messages cell to cell. They are not just limited to sexual functions. There are different types of hormones that regulate metabolism, digestion, growth, hunger and blood sugar (insulin). Hormone function and balance can be disrupted by toxins we take in, by foods we eat, and by natural age-related decline of the body, as with menopause. We still have a lot to learn about the loss of hormones in declining years, and still don't know everything about controlling the hormones related to most organs and functions. We do know some about those related to the male and female sexual functions: pregnenolone, DHEA, progesterone, estrogen, and testosterone. Still not precisely, but we've made great strides in controlling deficiencies and their side effects. Many factors besides age can affect hormone levels, such as stress, diet, drugs and toxins.

Many health concerns have been found to be connected with hormone deficiency, including depression, muscle pain, skin tone, insomnia, anxiety, libido, bone loss and memory. A complete hormone panel is recommended when any of these problems exist, and especially for anyone over 50.

Both men and women are subject to hormone deficiencies; testosterone in men fades libido, decreases muscle mass, and can affect the prostate.

Deficiencies can play a role in many diseases, including cancer, by the imbalance between hormones, such as high estrogen score without a high progesterone score. Pharmaceutical grade hormones (shots, gels) could have potential to increase the risk of health issues with side effects, while bio-identical hormone cream (not pills) have shown over time to be effective in increasing hormone levels that have declined with aging or hysterectomy, as long as the balance is addressed between all hormones, including thyroid. Hormones are yet another area where the balance between them is so critical. There are a few natural herbs, such as fenugreek extract (testofen), that may help push natural hormones through the system.

Cooking Tips to Improve Your Health

- Buy 'green' cooking pans to replace Teflon and aluminum pans
- Never cook on high heat
- Do not add garlic at the start of the cooking process.
- Add as many vegetables possible to dishes at every meal
- Add spice whenever possible, and as much as can be tasteful
- Rinse any foods marinated/packaged in white distilled vinegar
- Use raw honey for uncooked foods; regular honey for cooking
- Mix natural peanut butter with natural almond butter
- Boil meatballs (and other meats)

1. Cooking Pans

Most types of pots and pans have potential to leach metals or toxins into foods as they cook. At high heat, Teflon pans may release carcinogens and pollutants because of perfluorooctanoic acid (PFOA) used in the manufacture of Teflon cookware. This toxic chemical is set to be banned from all cookware by the year 2015. *'Green'* pans, called so because they are environmentally friendly, are void of this chemical, as well as another potentially toxic substance polytetrafluoroethylene (PTFE) with some.

Cooking acidic foods in aluminum pans will cause them to leach aluminum into foods. This factor has been implicated as a contributor to Alzheimer's disease. Anodized aluminum pans are made to assure that this does not happen, but imported aluminum pans are still suspect. Aluminum is considered a toxin by the U.S. Department of Health and Human Services.

Because copper can cause health problems, copper pans are generally coated with tin or stainless steel. Yet, tin cans are now lined because of health concerns due to leaching into foods, and that concern is passed on to tin lined pans. Adverse effects of cooking with stainless steel are negligible.

Cooking with certain ceramic cookware can pose a problem with lead. Imported ceramic pans are the least trusted, and should be avoided or researched. Also, ceramic cookware should not be placed in the dishwasher because the glaze can be worn down, and expose harmful chemicals underneath.

Green pans are generally made with a ceramic or silicone nonstick coating. Some are very non-stick at first use, but then food tends to stick more as they are used. The more reliable pans are made to last. There are many on the market to try, with new ones introduced all the time as the Teflon components are soon to be banned.

All types of cookware are still questionable and under scrutiny as each new type is introduced. We now have silicone baking pans, but they are really too new to judge their safety. Glass, ceramic, enamel and stainless steel are the best choices at the present time.

2. Cooking Heat

All foods can be cooked very well and deliciously on low heat; turn to high to get things going, and then place on low. Just like the speedometer in an automobile, it may read 180 miles per hour, but you never drive at that speed. As well, the dial on your stove should never be set on high -- more nutrients will be lost, flavors are actually diminished, and food molecules are detrimentally transformed.

Besides the loss of enzymes in cooking, there are several toxic elements created in cooking. This is especially important for cooking such foods as eggs and starchy foods like potatoes. Acrylamide for example is a natural substance that forms in any food that has been "browned", so to speak...the browning of toast, potatoes, meats, and even zucchini on a barbeque. This includes frying, deep-frying, toasting, barbequing, broiling, etc. It becomes a potentially toxic or cancer-causing substance as the food is browned. The darker the browning, and the more browned foods consumed, the more harm; especially true with breaded, deep-fried foods.

By keeping the cooking temperature low, it can lower the risk of acrylamide. Covering foods cooking on 'low' helps to retain the moisture, helps foods finish faster, more evenly, and moist. Keeping the skins on potatoes also helps.

Cooking on low heat can only increase the worth of cooking foods. Eggs are delicious covered and cooked on low heat. Foods take longer to cook, of course, but it's worth it. Since you will be changing your ways, and no longer cook on high heat, the *smoke factor* for cooking oils no longer is a concern; the biggest concern is the omega 3 content in oils exposed to heat. The omega 3 oils are very delicate and easily offended by high heat. In low temp cooking, the omega 3 content may be preserved. There are some cooking oils that should never be used for high-heat cooking, especially deep-frying.

3. Garlic

The medicinal nutrients within garlic are easily lost when cooked. It has shown to be as effective as prescription antibiotics, and effective in stopping candida. For nutritional benefit, always add garlic when you are done cooking the dish. For more of the wonderful garlic flavor, add either fresh garlic or garlic powder while you cook, then, when finished, mix in more freshly chopped garlic to reap its benefits.

4. Vegetables

Many people use simple ways in making a certain food dish or follow a recipe accordingly, but always keep an open mind to including additional vegetables that aren't listed in the recipe to any dish you may think is possible, and that could add more fiber and nutrients. In making spaghetti, try adding sliced onion, sliced zucchini or green peppers. In fixing eggs in the morning, try adding onions, tomatoes, mushrooms or spinach. Introduce vegetables into every meal...breakfast, lunch and dinner. With the addition of vegetables with every meal, the acidic effect of such foods as eggs, meats, rice, and bread can be diminished or counterbalanced by the alkaline effect of the vegetables.

5. Spices

Keep your imagination open for adding spices to dishes you may have not added before. Spices can add nutritional value to a meal. Spices add alkalinity along with micronutrients and antioxidants. In the case of curry, it is loaded with various antibiotic and liver cleansing spices such as turmeric, which is also a highly touted supplement used for warding off pain and cancer. Paprika, garlic, oregano are just a few of the flavorful spices that could be added into breakfast, lunch or dinner dishes. Remember, if not using fresh herbs, rehydrate the dried herbs in a small amount of water; this will bring out more flavor, and soften the texture of the herbs.

6. Vinegar

There are so many marinated food products drenched in white distilled vinegar made from grains, however this adds acidity to the foods. There is a difference of opinions among some professionals as to a gluten reaction from grain vinegars; some say gluten can come out of vinegar, some say there is not any concern. What I recognize as the biggest concern in vinegars is its acidic composition. I recommend to always rinse them off before eating to lower the acidic content. Always look for and choose foods marinated in apple cider vinegar instead, which benefits the body rather than working against it as with distilled vinegar. Its use as a marinade is rare, but in time I hope to see more manufacturers marinating foods in apple cider vinegar.

7. Honey

There is a misconception as to the benefits of commercial honey. Those touted benefits really belong to raw honey rather than the typical processed honey from the supermarket. Commercial honey is a great flavor enhancer, and should only be looked at for that reason. Most commercial honeys are pasteurized, killing so much of the nutritional content; it has a very high glycemic load (GL), while raw honey is about one-fourth lower. Other surprising facts about commercial honey include the fact that very often the honey you buy may not be pure honey; they are often mixed with cheaper sugars, even high fructose corn syrup. Some brands of honey are imported, and these are often mixed with sugars and flavoring. Even some fast food establishments dispense packets of altered honey. Always try to check for ingredients on the package or label.

It is the raw honey that possesses the medicinal qualities; it's great for burns, digestion and sore throats, and much more. Raw honey has more nutrients, but high heat will destroy its beneficial enzymes and nutrients. When cooking, use the inexpensive honey for flavor if need be, but if you want to add health benefits to your food, add it after the meal is cooked. It's great to spread onto toast with cinnamon for breakfast.

> *Side note: In my research, I have been disheartened in finding the fact that often some beekeepers feed their bees sugar...yes white refined sugar. This is done because their store of food has gone (the honey we take from them), and they need sustenance. My thought is that, just like feeding grains to farmed fish, bees are fed a substance that not only is not their regular diet, but it gets passed on to us.*

8. Mix natural peanut butter with natural almond butter

Peanut butter is a high inflammatory, acidic food. Peanuts do have good qualities; they are full of minerals, and the B vitamin content is higher than most nuts, but compared to almonds, they fall short in helping the body with alkalinity. Peanut oil has a high content of omega 6; almond oil has a higher omega 3, and is an alkaline food. Mixing the two gives the peanut flavor with added benefits from the almond, and helps cancel out the acidic effect.

9. Boil meatballs (and other meats)

There is no need to fry meatballs in oil anymore, and possibly other meat dishes. Just form the meatballs, bring a pan of water to a boil, and drop them in. Let boil for one minute, remove and drain; they become very firm, and hold up better than if they were fried in oil. Add meatballs to a pan of pasta sauce and cover to finish the cooking process. This avoids the heated oils that create free radicals, and the increase in toxic acrylamides that come with browning meat.

Healthful Kitchen Habits

- Refrigerate all oils, nuts, seeds
- Change plastic storage to glass
- Use several utensils during preparation/cooking to reduce contamination
- Never microwave frozen fruit or vegetables to defrost or cook
- Do not freeze bread products, nuts or coffee
- Microwave your cleaning sponges and dishrags daily
- Cutting Board Cleaning
- Wear gloves

1. Refrigerate oils, nuts, seeds

Refrigerate foods that have a high-content of oil, such as: cooking oils, omega 3 supplements, flaxseed, nuts, Vitamins A, D or E; any of these can become rancid, creating free radicals within the body. Rancidity occurs when oils are exposed to air, heat or light for a lengthy period of time, altering the fat molecules through oxidation. Rancid oil will smell funny. Storing oils in a cupboard above the stove has been a standing tradition, but the heat from the stove warms oils, and accelerates rancidity. Instead of gambling, it's safer to just refrigerate all oil. Hydrogenated oil was invented to allow oily foods, such as bakery goods, to be kept on the shelves or on kitchen counters for long periods of time, but this type of altered oil is a health hazard and must be avoided. Nuts and seeds have high contents of oil. These oils can become rancid from being housed in very warm places for too long, just like any bottled cooking oil can. And since packaged nuts at the supermarket can be warehoused and shelved for long periods of time, it is first important to smell the contents as soon as you open them to see if you can detect a rancid odor. If it smells funny, if it tastes odd, then return them to the market; it is not rare for this to happen.

Coconut and olive oils will solidify in the refrigerator. It's a good idea to put some olive oil in a glass container with a wide mouth so it can be scooped out as needed. Coconut oil hardens much more than olive oil, and is difficult to scoop. I suggest that a small amount at a time (one or two cups) be stored in a cool cupboard to be used as needed; coconut oil is much safer because it contains none of its natural enzymes, and rancidity does not occur as fast as other oils, just as it is safer to use in cooking.

Keep in mind, all oils will turn rancid over time, even when refrigerated. This starts from the day they are extracted, so it can also depend on how long they've been on the supermarket shelf.

Even Omega 3 oil supplements can become rancid when stored improperly. When shopping for an oil-based supplement, shake the container to see if the pills have clumped together. The pills should shake loosely inside. If you hear one big lump, then avoid it.

2. Change plastic storage to glass

Plastics have overwhelmingly found their way into kitchens, and it may be disrupting our hormone balance and health in many ways. From the supermarket to our refrigerator drawers, plastic is encasing what we eat. There are definite, legitimate warnings to never microwave foods in plastic containers because it contains a chemical prone to taint the food significantly when heated. Research has proven it goes even further than this. Milk packaged in glass bottles has shown to contain toxins from plastic as well, and the conclusion was made that the source was the soft flexible plastic tubing fitted around the cows' udders where the warm milk drains through.

Officials claim that all plastic used in food marketing and kitchen products stay at levels within safety limits where leaching is minimal. However, how much exposure does that include? When all the different limits of exposures are added up, and the lengths of time are calculated, is the exposure still safely within limits? We now live in a plastic world, and possibly if much of our food-related items can change from being plastic to glass or other non-chemical-leaching items, maybe our bodies would absorb fewer toxins. Most of this is out of our hands. Changing what we can might have some effect individually. Instead of plastic wrap, try using foil, paper towels, paper bags, waxed paper, ceramic or glass bowls, to do as much as you can to cut down on plastic exposure.

Think of all the ways our foods are exposed to plastics:

Plastic refrigerator drawers	*Plastic shopping bags*
Plastic cutting boards	*Plastic water bottles*
Plastic wrap	*Teflon cooking pans*
Plastic storage containers	*polytetrafluoroethylene (PTFE)*
Plastic storage bags	*Plastic mixing bowls*
Plastic packaging of meats	*Plastic mixing spoons*
Plastic packaging of frozen foods	*Plastic juice and milk containers*
Plastic knives	*Plastic margarine tubs*
Plastic microwave containers	*BPA in the lining of cans*
Plastic cooking oil bottles	

Begin saving the glass bottles and jars that prepared foods and drinks are packaged in, like dressings, sauces, mineral waters, etc., and build a supply for using as containers for leftovers, dressings and more, replacing the plastics. Glass containers are a precious commodity. Use a small club soda bottle for a nutritious homemade salad dressing that you can put in your purse or briefcase to carry out to a restaurant with you.

3. Utensils

When an eating utensil, such as a knife, is exposed to meats or other protein foods that easily spoil, DO NOT then expose it to a food container such as mayonnaise that does not spoil quickly. For example, cutting a piece of bologne, and then placing that knife in a jar of mayonnaise or mustard, which has a lengthy shelf-life, deposits the bacteria from the meat into the jar, and will become a bed of unhealthful bacteria. Cutting a pickle and then placing the knife in a jar of mayonnaise will not affect it because the pickle is filled with the natural preservative vinegar, and pickles do not spoil. Remember to change and use multiple knives as you prepare your meals with jarred or packaged products; this will cut down tremendously on stomach issues.

4. Microwave

Frozen, as do fresh, fruits and vegetables still have active natural enzymes, and microwaving these would eradicate those enzymes. Just place any frozen fruits and vegetables in a warm bowl of water to defrost, or place them in a bowl, put into the refrigerator before you go to bed, and the next morning they will be perfectly defrosted and ready to eat or use.

5. Freezing foods

Freezing breads, nuts and coffee has been a longtime tradition for preserving these food products. But this tradition started in the days when freezers were cooled by frozen ice. In today's modern world, freezers are cooled by an extremely different method because of wanting the *defrost* feature. Freezers today are cooled by actually pulling out the heat, leaving it void of hot air, and thus making the compartment cold. As this happens, the moisture in the foods in the freezer will also be pulled out. This is why you see frost on the inside of the wrappers of frozen foods. It's being pulled out and trapped by the wrapper. It used to be just the opposite; that the frost you would see would be on the outside of the wrapper, called "freezer burn". Here's how it is explained by a thermodynamics professional:

How Does a Freezer Work? *(Wisegeek.org)*

"A refrigerator does not cool items by lowering their original temperatures; instead, an evaporating gas called a refrigerant draws heat away, leaving the surrounding area much colder. Refrigerators and air conditioners both work on the principle of cooling through evaporation."

With this happening to your foods, taste is pulled out of the food along with the moisture, leaving you with, as time goes by, foods such as coffee, steak, bread or casseroles with less flavor, and a lot less moisture. In addition, the refrigerator section maintains its coolness in the same manner, only at a much slower rate. It makes more sense to store breads, nuts, coffee, etc., in the refrigerator. But for the foods that do spoil in a matter of days such as meats, casseroles, etc., they do need to be in the freezer, and using them as soon as possible will save them from dehydration and loss of taste. Foods stored in the freezer for months will turn out to be dry and tasteless.

6. Cleaning sponges, cleaning cloths

Germs and bacteria in the kitchen are always a problem, and one common source is the dishrag or sponge that's used to clean dishes and counters. Microwaving these things for at least 1 minute will kill the germs and bacteria before and/or after you use them. A hot dishwasher will also help, but changing your rags and sponges daily is the optimum solution.

7. Cleaning cutting boards

Cutting boards must be disinfected after or before every use. It is not good enough to have one cutting board for meats and one for other foods. Think about it; if you do cut meat, that cutting board needs to be disinfected enough to kill all contaminating germs, in order to use that board once again in the future even if you are again cutting meat. It's mostly a matter of when you are cutting what. If you are cutting meat and vegetables for your dinner meal, it certainly doesn't matter because you will be eating both for dinner. If you are cutting meat for lunch, and then cutting raw vegetables to store in the refrigerator, then it does matter. So it makes perfect sense to cut the vegetables first and then the meat. But to say you need different boards for different foods is not necessary.

No matter what, all cutting boards need to be disinfected; here is what works: *extremely* hot water, borax, white vinegar, lemon juice, hydrogen peroxide, or combinations thereof. Last resort is bleach water.

8. Wear gloves

Surgical gloves, or the like, are great for preparing foods. They are great for handling meats; the juices and fat residue will stay away from under the fingernails, and the need to wash hands will be kept at a minimum. They can be tossed after preparing meat. Changing gloves for different stages of meal preparation is a good practice for controlling contamination.

Recipe Replacements

This list shows how you can replace common, unhealthful ingredients with substitutes that are non-dairy, lower glycemic load, alkaline instead of acid, and more nutritious.

Common Ingredient		Replacement Ingredient
Agave	=	Coconut Sugar Nectar, Raw Honey (*cold recipes only*)
Breadcrumbs	=	Use sprouted grain bread to make breadcrumbs (saving the end pieces works well); Break bread into small pieces, lay onto cookie sheet, bake at 190 until dry. (about 20 minutes) crumble/pound into crumbs

Brown Sugar	=	Sucanat or coconut sugar (each 1:1 ratio)
Buttermilk	=	Coconut milk (any alternative milk) 1 TBLS apple cider vinegar per cup. Let ferment together for 15 minutes before using
Chocolate Square	=	Raw cocoa powder, unsweetened; 3 TBLS cocoa plus 1 TBLS butter/oil equals 1 square of dark unsweetened chocolate (one ounce)
		Chocolate sauce: add 1 TBLS xylitol with 2 tsp coconut sugar, and 1 TBLS coconut milk (or more, according to how thick you need it)
Cornstarch	=	Whole grain flours; arrowroot 2:1 (cannot be boiled; add at end of cooking time
Cream	=	Cashew milk (find in recipe chapter)
Egg whites	=	Free Range, Whole Eggs; when recipes call for only yolks, use whites for meringue or something else; if recipes call for only whites, use yolks for sauces, puddings, etc., but always try to incorporate the yolk or white into an accompanying food dish product.
Flours	=	Use any whole grains: wheat, brown rice, coconut, oat, almond, quinoa, amaranth, millet; combine any grains for different textures and flavors. Self-rising, all-purpose, etc., are unnecessary in healthy cooking.
Honey	=	For cooking, use regular honey (gives flavor only); for non-cooked recipes such as salad dressings, use raw honey (gives nutritional benefits); or add raw honey when a cooked dish has finished cooking, before serving. Coconut sugar nectar also a substitute.

Lard	=	See Vegetable Oil entry below
Margarine	=	*Canola Harvest*, *Good Balance*, Olive Oil, Coconut oil, Flaxseed oil, homemade margarine (see Recipes), grass-fed butter
Milk	=	Coconut or cashew milk for cooking, baking, sauces, etc./almond, hemp, brown rice, oat, flax milk for non-cooked recipes
Oil & Vinegar Salad Dressing	=	Extra virgin olive oil with balsamic, fresh lemon juice, apple cider vinegar or red wine vinegar (spices)
Powdered Sugar	=	1 cup xylitol and 2 TBLS arrowroot; blend on high for 20 seconds; (Sucanat can be used)
Rice Vinegar	=	Brown rice vinegar
Salt	=	Sea Salt
Vegetable Oil	=	Look for and use any expeller-pressed, cold-pressed, or virgin oils only Non-cooked foods: Flaxseed For cooking: Olive, high-oleic sunflower, coconut *(sesame and peanut are high in omega 6, so limit to occasional specialty meals (Asian dish), would be okay)* Corn and grapeseed oils are extremely high in omega 6, so I recommend not using them ***For added nutrition, replace at least 1/4 oil in any recipe with coconut oil*
Distilled Vinegar	=	Apple cider vinegar (unfiltered)
Whipped Cream	=	Coconut Milk (See recipe chapter)
White Sugar	=	Xylitol (1:1) , erythritol (1:2) , Stevia (20:1) Luo Han (25:1) *(hard to find in pure form,)*

Supermarket Purchasing Tips

1. READ THE INGREDIENTS
2. READ THE INGREDIENTS
3. READ THE INGREDIENTS

I want to say this over and over, because this is the most important thing to do in purchasing food and eating healthfully; it can't be said enough. The list of ingredients on labels should be looked at first before purchasing packaged foods. Ingredients are listed by quantity, so any foods that list sugars at the beginning should be avoided. Look for all sugars (see list below), hydrogenated ingredients, nitrites, and any words that are unfamiliar or can't be pronounced. 'Natural flavor' is just one way manufacturers have license to slip in unhealthy ingredients unsuspectingly.

Nutrition Facts

Serving Size 244 g

Amount Per Serving	
Calories 168	Calories from Fat 89

	% Daily Value*
Total Fat 10g	16%
Saturated Fat 7g	33%
Trans Fat	
Cholesterol 27mg	9%
Sodium 122mg	5%
Total Carbohydrate 11g	4%
Dietary Fiber 0g	0%
Sugars 11g	
Protein 9g	

Vitamin A	10%	Vitamin C	5%
Calcium	33%	Iron	1%

*Percent Daily Values are based on a 2,000 calorie diet. Your daily values may be higher or lower depending on your calorie needs.

NutritionData.com

In looking at the "Nutrition Facts" box on packaging, the amount of sodium, protein and fiber are the most important facts listed. If it's a fruit product, the sugar content noted will be deceptive, because fruit is basically all sugar, and therefore it will list as having a very high sugar content anyway. That's why it's most important to view the ingredients instead of "Nutrition Facts", and look for all forms of sugar.

Here is the list of ingredients for a popular "whole wheat" English muffin:

Whole Wheat Flour, Water, **Honey**, **Brown Sugar**, **Rice Flour**, Yeast, **Wheat Gluten**, Whole Flaxseed, **Soybean Oil**, Cornmeal, Salt, Calcium Propionate (Preservative) Monoglycerides, **DATEM**, Potassium Sorbate, **Modified Cornstarch, Soy Protein**, Ascorbic Acid.

Notice in bold lettering the sugars (honey, brown sugar), refined ingredients (rice flour, cornstarch), wheat gluten, and refined soy products (soybean oil, soy protein), all of which are counter-nutrients. This reveals that a *whole wheat* product does not mean it is healthful.

One big negative of eating out at restaurants rather than cooking at home is the fact that there are no labels and lists of ingredients that can be inspected. It's always a mystery as to what is in any restaurant meal. By cooking at home, we have choices in what goes into our meals.

Commercial Everyday Foods Containing Added Sugar (or sugar substitutes) that can easily be avoided

READ LABELS AT ALL TIMES

The sugars added in foods are often unnoticed by the consumer, and by reading the ingredients, and finding alternative products or brands that do not include sugar, the added sugar can *easily* be avoided and eliminated from your daily diet. Here are popular food products that can contain added sugars, and do have alternative brands that do not have it:

- Sodas/Flavored Waters/Milks
- Tomato products: Spaghetti Sauce, Salsa, Stewed Tomatoes, Ketchup, Tomato Sauce
- Applesauce
- Peanut Butter
- Yogurt
- Jelly/Jam
- Fruit Juices
- Cereals

Just by avoiding sugar in these products alone, your daily sugar intake will substantially reduce, aiding a lower blood sugar count, fewer blood sugar spikes, and a decrease in inflammation. The average sugar intake of the average American is about 156 pounds per year. This amount includes the many additive sugars in everyday products.

These items can just as well be purchased without sugar by changing brands; simply, READ THE INGREDIENTS ON THE LABEL. Sugars are found in an abundance of ready-made products; all these small sugar sources add up to a continuous flow of sugar through the body daily, contributing to the onset of diabetes, high blood pressure, weight gain and various health problems.

The higher content of sugar listed on a label, the more inflammatory effect, and the higher effect on blood insulin. Alkaline sugars, noted with asterisks, tend to have anti-inflammatory effects, with less effect on blood sugar.

Sugar comes in many forms by many names; here is a list (*the more acceptable forms have an asterisk*):

Acesulfame K Potassium

Agave

Aspartame (Equal, Nutrasweet)

Barley malt*

Brown Rice Syrup*

Brown Sugar

Erithrytol*

Evaporated cane juice

Fructose

Fruit juice

Galactose

Glucose

High fructose corn syrup

Honey*

Inulin*

Lactose

Luo Han*

Malt

Maltodextrin

Maltose

Cane juice crystals

Caramel

Corn sweetener

Cornstarch

Corn syrup

Dextrin

Mannitol*

Maple syrup*

Molasses*

Raw Honey*

Rice syrup

Saccharin (Sweet' n Low)

Stevia*

Sucanat*

Sucralose (Splenda)

Sucrose

Treacle

Turbinado

Xylitol*

1. Sodas/Flavored Waters/Alternative Milks

Everyone is aware of the fact that the main ingredient in soft drinks is sugar. But since sugar was found to contain calories that made people fat, the food industry introduced the sugar substitutes that contained little or no calories. It has been discovered that the body doesn't care that it is calorie free, the body still understands it is a "sugar", and therefore the pounds still pile on. This chemically altered sugar plays a trick on the brain. Plus, the 'altered sugar substitutes' (the calorie-free sweeteners like Sucralose) are chemically mutated products that wreak havoc in the system. Besides not keeping the weight off, they are jeopardizing the health of those who ingest them. Water is the best, most natural alternative.

By reading the guidelines within this book, it's noted that even commercial fruit juices should be avoided because they are in themselves a refined sugar product that contributes to arterial inflammation. The ingredients on flavored waters should be read to make sure of their content because you can't rely on their name; some have just a mild natural fruit flavoring, while others are full-blown sugar water.

The non-dairy milks on the market, such as almond milk, rice milk, soymilk, all come in unsweetened and sweetened varieties. Always look for and choose the variety that is UNSWEETENED. If it says "original", "natural", or anything other than unsweetened, you can be assured it will contain a sugar of some kind.

2. Tomato Products: Spaghetti Sauce/Salsa/Stewed Tomatoes

There are several commercial spaghetti sauces that do not have added sugar, and they taste as good or better; again, read the ingredients on the label. For one, Costco's Kirkland Marinara sauces are without sugar and very tasty. There are great salsas made without sugar, and, if you can, find one without *white/distilled vinegar* as well, possibly with apple cider vinegar or lime juice. Stewed tomatoes should be avoided because they invariably contain added sugar. The nature of "stewed tomatoes" is that they are sweetened. To find an un-sugared tomato product, always READ THE LIST OF INGREDIENTS ON THE LABEL.

3. Applesauce

Applesauce is one food that definitely does not need the added sugar to taste good, and yet manufacturers seem to think they do. Natural, unsweetened applesauce has a great taste, and is even better with added cinnamon. Cinnamon lowers blood sugar, blood pressure and triglycerides, and is great for combating diabetes. To find an un-sugared applesauce, READ THE LIST OF INGREDIENTS ON THE LABEL. Since commercial processed applesauce has no enzymes or peel, fresh apples or homemade applesauce are the best options.

4. Peanut Butter

Most commercial peanut butters, even the top brands, may have added sugar PLUS homogenized oil. The main reason people shy away from *natural* peanut butter is the fact that pure peanut butter has a natural separation of the peanut oil and the peanut mass, which needs to be mixed together before being used. It takes but one minute to mix and refrigerate. Once stored in the refrigerator, it will hold its melded consistency. The hydrogenation process used in making the popular peanut butters causes it to gel together, not allowing it to separate at room temperature. Hydrogenated oil is similar to trans fat; the molecules are altered, and it will cause inflammation in the body. True oil-containing products such as peanut butter should be refrigerated to deter rancidity, and the hydrogenated oils do not because, healthwise, they are already beyond rancidity. To make sure you are buying the pure peanut butter, READ THE LIST OF INGREDIENTS ON THE LABEL. It will merely list: peanuts and salt.

5. Yogurt

Yogurt is known for its probiotic ingredient, acidophillis. A probiotic is good for the body because it will help equalize the good and the bad bacteria within the gut. Adding sugar or fruit to yogurt defeats the main purpose of yogurt because it is a main source of food that feeds the bad bacteria, so you are actually feeding your bad bacteria as you are trying to eradicate it. There are several commercial yogurts that do not have added sugar. Look for the yogurts called "plain", but just in case, still READ THE LIST OF INGREDIENTS ON THE LABEL.

6. Jellies/Jams

Most commercial jams and jellies are made with sugar, and it's a misconception that they have to be made with sugar. There are a few brands on the market that are made without refined sugar or sugar substitutes. To find an un-sugared jam or jelly, READ THE LIST OF INGREDIENTS ON THE LABEL. St. Dalfour and Smucker's are brands that make jams and jellies without sugar.

7. Fruit Juice

Commercial fruit juices are basically sweet enough without adding refined or sugar substitutes to them, but some makers do, adding fuel to the fire. One of the most outrageously deceptive, unhealthful products to come along is one that is marketed as something good for your kids. Here are its ingredients:

> Water, **High Fructose**, **Corn Syrup** and 2% or Less of Each of the Following: Concentrated Juices (Orange, Tangerine, Apple, Lime, Grapefruit). Citric Acid, Ascorbic Acid (Vitamin C), Beta-Carotene, Thiamin Hydrochloride (Vitamin B1), Natural Flavors, **Food Starch-Modified**, **Canola Oil**, Cellulose Gum, Xanthan Gum, **Sodium Hexametaphosphate**, Sodium Benzoate To Protect Flavor, **Yellow #5, Yellow #6**

Besides only containing 2% fruit juice, it is mostly high fructose and corn syrup, with the added yellow dyes, also known as tartrazine, which are a major cause of allergies and hyperactivity in children. Sodium Hexametaphosphate has potential irritant effects on the kidneys.

8. Cereals

It's almost impossible to find a cereal product that does not contain sugar in some form. Very many contain evaporated cane juice, honey, brown sugar, etc. But also the typical cereal itself is refined and speeds through the system, and increases the insulin response. This reaction not only increases body fat, but it also has been proven to potentially stimulate tumor growth. Safe whole-grain cereals include: puffed brown rice, puffed millet, oatmeal, amaranth, quinoa (hot or cold), and sprouted grain varieties – all void of added sugars.

Worst Foods to Purchase

- Soft Drinks/Diet drinks/Fruit Juices/Energy Drinks
- Farmed salmon, and other farmed fish
- Restaurant breakfasts
- Artificial sweeteners
- Potato Chips/French Fries
- White Bread/phony 'wheat' bread
- Canned Foods
- Bagged microwave popcorn

1. Soft Drinks/Diet drinks/Fruit Juices/Energy Drinks

It cannot be stressed enough how these drinks have infiltrated our diets, and contributed to every one of our top diseases in America. Any of these bottled drinks is just sugared water, pure and simple. Most of the flavored water drinks must be checked for any sugar ingredients; names can be deceptive. Even the plain fruit juices of any kind must be viewed as a sugar drink because it invariably contains none of the natural fiber intended to slow the insulin effect of the juice running through the bloodstream. It is basically high fructose, the sugar substance we need to keep to a minimum. Energy drinks include high caffeine; diet drinks include the artificial sweeteners; and many drinks include color dyes.

2. Farmed salmon, and other farmed fish

It is constantly proclaimed that salmon is one of the most nutritious foods a person can eat. It is full of omega 3, anti-inflammatory elements, and packed full of nutrients. And this is all true. Except for one thing. Farmed salmon is unfortunately the complete opposite. Farmed salmon is as bad for you as wild salmon is good for you. Farmed salmon, because it is corralled with thousands of other salmon, are injected with toxic antibiotics to help keep them from catching and spreading infections; salmon farms act as breeding grounds for parasitic sea lice, they are given growth hormones to fatten them up; they are fed grains which fatten them up, instead of the natural diet of krill and other natural sea foods that wild salmon eat. All this contributes to inflammation in the body. Then as the fish mature, because of all these unnatural processes they are subjected to, their skin color turns a grey color instead of the bright pinkish orange of wild salmon; and so they are then given dye, another toxin. And even with the dye, the color of the salmon becomes a pale pink, rather than the luscious bright pinkish orange of wild salmon. Put them side by side and you will see the difference.

3. Restaurant breakfasts

For some reason, breakfast has turned into a sugar feast: pancakes, crepes, Danish, coffeecakes, and waffles with chocolate chips, caramel, and topped with whipped cream and pure sugar syrup. But the overall breakfast menus are also filled with highly refined grains (toast, muffins, bagels, pancakes, waffles, cereals), plus high fat (steaks, ham, sausage and bacon). Yogurts and even fruits have sugar added, cheese often tops the potatoes. The oils used to cook eggs and potatoes are suspect, and are very likely either hydrogenated or inexpensive high omega 6, which contribute to arthritis, joint pain, and more.

4. Artificial sweeteners

The public was thrown a curve when artificial sweeteners were introduced as a 'no calorie' alternative to sugar. It sucked millions into this false claim of keeping weight off. Since losing weight is the number one concern with people and their eating, they bought it, and have held on tightly to their cans of diet soda. However, it's been proven that these sweeteners actually do just the opposite; they cause the brain to think that the appetite has not been satiated, and needs more food, and so defeats its intended purpose. Because of its chemical makeup, the consequences are more a concern than common sugar.

5. Potato Chips/French Fries

Potatoes are not basically bad for you. But take that potato, remove the peel, and deep fry it at high heat, especially in a hydrogenated oil, and it will cause great damage to your system. It is both the high heat and the trans fat that they are drenched in that render the potato unhealthful. Potatoes, more than most foods, contain acrylamide, a cancer-causing chemical, that when fried, broiled or baked at very high temperatures will release its negative impact.

6. White Bread/phony 'whole wheat' bread

Common white refined flour is overly pervasive in our society, and we need to stop eating it. Ninety percent of the breads sold in the supermarkets are junk. They are refined, whether they say whole grain or not; most have added sugars, hydrogenated oils. *Flour* is refined grain. Just because it says whole wheat does not mean it is 100% whole grain. The law allows the description of *whole grain* as long as the grain ingredients are at least 51% whole grain. This leaves 49% that can be refined white grain. The best and only breads to purchase are 100% sprouted grain breads. For one thing, having this at home will help balance in some respect what you are getting in the restaurants.

7. Canned Foods

Canned foods were developed for the days before adequate distribution of foods to far off places, but we are no longer dependent on canned foods. Purchasing canned fruits and vegetables should be the last resort. The contents are pasteurized, losing their enzymes; and way too much sugars and salt are added. Now there is the threat of the carcinogenic chemical BPA that is in the inner lining of most cans. Fresh and frozen fruits and vegetables are the only types to purchase. Some canned meats and beans in non-BPA cans are acceptable.

8. Pre-Bagged microwave popcorn

Contained in the buttery flavored additive in pre-bagged microwave popcorn is an ingredient called diacetyl. Scientists have found that this substance is linked to respiratory problems, and may pose a risk in the development of Alzheimer's disease by causing increased clumping of a certain protein in the brain. Most buttery flavorings consist of hydrogenated oils, which are known to cause inflammation in the arteries.

PFOA (Perfluorooctanoic acid) is a chemical found in the lining of the popcorn bags. It is a known carcinogen, and is the same harmful chemical found in Teflon pans. This chemical enters the body both by fumes from the heated product and from ingesting it with the popcorn.

Both the diacetyl and PFOA have been under review for several years by the FDA, and studies have concluded detrimental health issues, yet they are still on the market. Because of a class-action lawsuit with Dupont, the manufacturer of PFOA has agreed to end production by 2015. For now, we are legally subjected to PFOA for more years.

Easy Between-Meals Snacks

- Any raw vegetables
- Popcorn
- Chocolate or berry shake
- Nuts and seeds
- Pickles, olives, marinated chili peppers, artichoke hearts
- Hummus w/brown rice crackers
- Baked plantain chips

Keep a lot of these nutritious snacks handy all day long for any cravings.

1. Any raw vegetables

Here are some new ideas other than carrot and celery sticks:

> Asparagus – this vegetable is actually crispy and tasty
> Sweet potato – cut them like carrot sticks
> Radishes – cut off the ends, and keep in a bowl of cool water
> Peppers, green, red, yellow, orange – cut into slices
> Snow peas – remove the stem and vein along the side
> Jicama – peeled or unpeeled, cut in strips, keep in cool water

All of these are full of fiber, and are alkaline.

2. Popcorn, air-popped, stove-top popped, or microwave, plain or w/olive oil, margarine/homemade margarine

Even though popcorn is a somewhat inflammatory food, it is however far less inflammatory than any other mainstream commercial chips and crackers. Buy the plain, uncooked popcorn kernels, and cook them either in an air-popping machine, in the microwave in a paper bag, or in a pan on the stove w/a little oil. Buy only organic (non-GMO also).

Popcorn is good fiber.

3. Chocolate or berry shake

For a pick-me-up snack, make a fruit or chocolate shake in the blender. Make it the night before or in the morning to keep on hand. (Recipes in the recipe chapter.)

Great for additional antioxidant nutrition.

4. Nuts and seeds

Bowls of nuts and seeds can be left out for easy access, easy snacking throughout the day. Doesn't matter what kind of nuts or seeds, as long as they are not sugared and drenched in hydrogenated oils. Buy natural nut butters to spread onto 100% whole grain crackers.

Healthful oils and fiber.

5. Dill pickles, olives, marinated chili peppers, artichoke hearts

These are all better choices than the usual junk food treats that most people munch on all day. Most of these are marinated in white vinegar, so I suggest they be rinsed before eating to cut down on the acid, unless they were marinated in apple cider vinegar; forget the sugared sweet pickles.

Good fiber, and alkaline vegetables

6. Hummus w/brown rice crackers

Hummus is basically a healthful dip or treat. It should consist of chickpeas/garbanzo beans, olive oil, tahini (sesame seed paste), garlic and lemon juice. (See recipe chapter.) Keep this on hand in your refrigerator, and eat with 100% brown rice or whole grain crackers, or fresh raw vegetables like those listed above.

Good fiber and protein

7. Baked plantain chips

Baked plantain chips can be found online, at Trader Joe's or other specialty shops. These are actually not sweet, but rather they taste more like potato chips than anything else, and are a good substitute for those addicted to potato chips.

Good fiber, and satisfies the chip quality of snacks

Top Restaurant Foods Not to Trust

- Salmon
- Whole-Wheat Bread
- Salad Dressings/Cooking Oils
- Eggs
- Sauces
- Butter/Margarine

Most restaurants are not health conscious, let's face it. They may try to purport that they are in some ways, but most often their ways will backfire on you. Restaurants want your return business, and the best way to do that is to make foods as tasty as possible with added salt, sugar or MSG, and at the same time offer the least expensive products to save dollars on their end. These following restaurant items are the most detrimental to your health.

1. Salmon

Be cautious in eating salmon at a restaurant. Restaurants want to provide customers with the number one selling fish on the market, but on the most part they will serve farmed salmon because of expense. You cannot trust a waitress/waiter to inform you whether the salmon is *farm raised* or *wild* if the menu doesn't indicate. Those who really know are the owner and chef. There is a possibility that even if you ask, the true answer may not be told by a waiter who does not really know the true answer. Or, even if it states "fresh", fresh does not mean wild. If the menu states wild, then it is most likely wild. However, I still remain skeptical. Ask to see a piece of the raw salmon before ordering it, or speak to the chef. The color of raw salmon is the best indicator between wild and farmed.

2. Whole Wheat Bread

The biggest misnomer in restaurants is the term *whole wheat* bread. The restaurant workers ask if you want white or wheat bread. First of all, *white* bread *is* wheat bread; there is no difference.

Whole wheat bread is one of the most misused terms in the restaurant industry. The truth is that manufacturers can label their bread whole wheat as long as it has included a minimum of 51% whole grain. The rest can be refined white flour, unbeknown to the consumer. If the package is labeled 100% whole grain bread, then it must be 100% whole grain only. The manufacturer of the 100% *whole wheat* bread has to adhere to the rule in packaging, but the restaurant does not.

All restaurants know they now need an option of whole-wheat bread to satisfy customers; unfortunately, some restaurants will buy the 'brown' colored basic wheat bread (colored with molasses), camouflaged to look "whole wheat", in order to save money. Besides, many people truly are fooled that because it looks brownish, and because it is called whole wheat, they believe it is 100% whole wheat, which it is not. And most of the time it's not even 51% whole grain. There are very few restaurants that truly serve 100% whole wheat bread because of the expense. If they do, they are truly looking out for the customer, and that is the restaurant to frequent. In eating out, I recommend you limit your consumption of bread, or, better yet, not have any at all. I know they put baskets of bread on the table, and it is the most difficult thing to reject; it's a true test.

3. Salad Dressings

It's difficult to find a *healthful* salad dressing in a restaurant. Here are the major popular dressings and the reasons they are usually unhealthful:

Oil & Vinegar

We tend to believe that oil and vinegar is one of the safest, most nutritious salad dressing choices to choose in a restaurant. At least we think so. The component of oil we usually assume would and should be used is olive; however, don't assume it is. The less exclusive the restaurant, the less concern about what oil is in a dressing. It could very well be just a salad oil like hydrogenated soybean. Restaurants use quite a bit of oil for cooking, and because of this they want to use the least expensive oil they can buy, for deep frying, etc. Some restaurants will use the same oil for salads as they use for deep frying. The health component of vinegar is usually never considered by the restaurant, but white vinegar is most commonly used. This is the least healthful of the vinegars. The better choices are the balsamic or red wine, and at the top of the list would be apple cider vinegar or lemon juice, but these are rarely considered. Even when served in the cruet, you may be getting lesser quality oils. Also, many of these restaurant oils are not refrigerated, leaving them vulnerable to rancidity, especially if stored in a warm kitchen.

Ranch

The most popular of salad dressings in America is the ranch dressing, and there is a simple reason for it – MSG (monosodium glutamate); it is a flavor enhancer that has addictive and allergenic qualities as well. The number one selling bottled dressing includes MSG, as do very many restaurant brands. MSG is used to enhance the food enough to make you want more; that's the only reason. Ranch dressing should be avoided, except you can find some without MSG if you look hard and read ingredients. Most brands of ranch dressing could also contain white vinegar, sugar, and plenty of chemicals; often hydrogenated oils, corn syrup, high fructose corn syrup, or fructose are used.

MSG is a very common additive for foods in Asian restaurants, but most of us are not aware that a vast majority of other types of restaurants use MSG in their foods as well. MSG is a known allergen, which can cause, in some people, headaches, migraines, rashes, hypertension, and may affect breathing in those with asthma. In addition, most fast-food restaurants are suspected of using MSG in their foods, but it is not easy to know what foods in what restaurants it is found in.

On the labels of foods we buy in grocery stores, MSG can also be listed as autolyzed yeast extract, hydrolyzed vegetable protein or HVP, potassium glutamate, sodium caseinate, broth, natural flavorings, or simply flavorings.

Vinaigrette

Vinaigrette dressings are usually a sweeter dressing compared to the simple mix of oil and vinegar, and reasoning tells you that, yes, sugar most likely has been added. Again the type of oil and type of vinegar used should be questioned.

Blue Cheese

The different brands of blue cheese dressings could include corn syrup, sugar, sodium nitrite, maltodextrin, distilled vinegar, cultured dextrose. Besides being a dairy product, blue cheese dressings have far too many unnecessary negative additives.

4. Eggs

Eggs are highly nutritious naturally, but in the restaurant business, there are various types of eggs that can be procured to make the preparation of eggs easier and *safer* for them. The first is the ready-made scrambled egg mix that comes in refrigerated cartons. Other forms are ready-made omelettes or egg "patties" that come frozen or refrigerated. All of which are pasteurized, and some possibly include preservatives. Also, the regular uncracked eggs can be bought pasteurized, eradicating the natural enzymes they would naturally contain. Restaurants are more prone to buying pasteurized/irradiated (treated with radiation) eggs for liability reasons. So eggs in any form served in a restaurant is suspect of not being natural, or may have such additives as corn syrup, artificial flavorings, corn oil and preservatives. I choose to have breakfast at home, but when eating out, the poached egg is the safest.

5. Sauces

The more delicious and flavorful the sauce that covers your meal, the more possibility of it containing an abundance of sugar, salt, hydrogenated oils or possibly MSG. Sauces are a big part of restaurant presentation and taste, but they come with the price of adding to heart disease.

6. Margarine

The commonly used brands of margarine used in restaurants still contain trans fat, or hydrogenated oils. Many restaurants use the less expensive brands of margarines in their cooking since no one is the wiser. The better restaurants will serve real butter (usually served in foil). There are very few restaurants that will use or serve the newer soft margarines made without trans fat. If you can have the choice of butter or margarine, take the butter, unless you know they can offer a margarine without hydrogenated oils. One thing we do not get to see is the kind of oils or margarines used in the kitchens. Do they really use real butter? Toasted bread that is delivered to your table could very well be hydrogenated margarine. Hydrogenated oils and margarines are most likely used in the cooking process for two reasons: 1) because it is cheaper to use, and 2) because trans fat creates better looking, better textured, and yes, better tasting foods in some cases. Health is not a top concern in most restaurant kitchens; it is taste and presentation.

Changes Needed by Food Providers

Restaurants and food manufacturers are listening and watching for clues as to what the public wants. There is some buzz from the public for more healthful items, but not enough and not fast enough. Restaurants should not wait until their patrons tell them to change, because most will go on eating the same junk foods they've expected. But some things can be changed without anyone really knowing; after all, look at how much added junk and additives goes into our food without us knowing and approving just in the grocery store products. But there are very many new options that can be offered for anyone's sake of wanting to eat healthier intentionally.

Here are just a few simple things that could be accomplished sooner than later, that would cut down on poor nutritional substances going into everyone's body; these simple changes could eliminate thousands of cases of obesity in America.

What Restaurants Need to Change for Better Health of their Patrons

- Offer Wild Salmon, help boycott farmed

- Do not use yogurt that contains sugar
- Leave out added sugar for most fruit drinks and fruit items
- Do not use hydrogenated oils
- Offer **100%** whole grain or sprouted grain breads, rolls, tortillas and buns, and without sugars or hydrogenated oils
- Offer more choices WITHOUT cheese
- Stop selling or using products with the ingredient High Fructose Corn Syrup (HFCS)
- Offer salad dressings that do not contain HFCS, sugar or hydrogenated oils
- Stop using hydrogenated oils for frying or in recipes
- Do not use powdered, processed, irradiated eggs
- Do not use MSG
- Change from using Canola or soy oil to Sunflower oil

What <u>Food Manufacturers</u> Need to Change for Better Health of the Public

- Do not include hydrogenated oils in products
- Do not include high fructose corn syrup in products
- Make all 100% whole grain or sprouted grain breads, rolls, tortilla and buns without sugars or hydrogenated oils
- Do not add MSG to products
- Change from using Canola or soy oil to Sunflower oil, coconut oil
- Eliminate the use of carrageenan as an additive to alternative milks
- Eliminate dyes in foods, as well as pet food.

And much more

Most Underrated Foods

- Eggs
- Potatoes
- Sweet Potatoes
- Nuts
- Shellfish
- Avocados
- Sardines
- Coconut

Most of these foods get a bad rap because they are thought to be either "fattening" or "unhealthy". The facts should be presented so more people can reap the benefits of these foods.

1. Eggs

Eggs do contain an exceptional amount of cholesterol. However, facts reveal that our liver produces about 70% of our body's cholesterol, and as our brain signals that we have the right amount floating through our system, then cholesterol production is halted. The brain is made up of about 80% cholesterol. When you see a picture of a brain with all its entangled ropes of woven fat globules, it consists of mostly cholesterol. Hormone production originates from cholesterol. In other words, our body needs cholesterol. Cholesterol is naturally floating in our blood at all times because it has its own necessary functions. Our bodies do not 'collect' cholesterol and dump it into our arteries; cholesterol from food gets processed through digestion just like any other food; but if this food-sourced cholesterol becomes *oxidized* by high-heat cooking, then the body views it as foreign matter, it's attacked, and the inflammation begins. If scarring of the arteries develops through inflammation, our natural cholesterol is called upon to help repair those arteries, thus providing a Band-Aid. This is one way we can develop plaque. This is why it's important to keep oxidation at a minimum when cooking cholesterol-sourced foods, especially eggs. Eggs contain a high amount of phosphatidylcholine, which is a substance that naturally breaks down cholesterol in digestion. This is one way an egg is actually helping with its own digestion. Eggs should be slow-cooked on low heat, without the yolk contacting the pan.

2. Potatoes

Because of the current diabetes and obesity epidemics in our society, and the need to monitor the glycemic load in foods, potatoes have declined in favor and popularity, even though they are full of nutrients; they contain more potassium than bananas, are a good source of Vitamin C, and as much fiber as whole grain bread. Russet potatoes have more potassium, phosphorus, magnesium and niacin than broccoli, and more fiber, choline and iron than zucchini. There is a higher consumption in central Europe than in the U.S.

It's been a misrepresentation that the starch in potatoes will put on weight; it's all in the way they are prepared, and we've abused them horribly by deep-frying, removing the skins, and piling on cheese, milk, salt and ketchup. Potatoes actually are comprised of an amount of resistant starch, which means it does not get digested right away. And if the potato is cooked then cooled, this will almost double the amount of resistant starch. Eating a potato with the skin gives an alkaline benefit; without the skin, it is acidic. Potatoes have one of the highest contents of phenols, which are powerful antioxidants, and have been found to possess antibacterial, antiviral, anti-inflammatory effects.

Starch is not a bad thing; it creates glucose, which is our body's primary source of energy. All starches and sugars are converted into glucose. An occasional simple baked potato with chicken stock, maybe a small amount of a nutritious oil or limited butter, and accompanied by nutritious vegetables, could be a worthwhile complement to any diet.

Starch has a way of making us feel full, which can be a good thing. Eating a side portion of starch will keep our cravings down between meals, whether its brown rice, potato or whole grains. Potatoes are a natural food, and weight gain comes with refined and/or abused starchy foods like French fries. Consuming potatoes at a few meals each week does not jeopardize health.

Almost any food has its negatives, and two negative aspects of the potato are its acrylamide and solanine content. When baked, broiled or fried at very high heat, the natural chemical acrylamide is accelerated (true with most foods); the more 'browning' occurring on the potato, the more acrylamide is present. This has been shown to be a potential carcinogenic. It's best to boil, steam, or cook on very low heat slowly to try to avoid as much of this natural chemical as possible. Just to point out, potatoes are not the only food with this natural chemical. It is in grains (when crust is browned), and in roasted coffee beans. And surprisingly, there is very high amount in chicory, which is a well-known coffee substitute.

Cut potatoes, rinse, soak in a pan of water for about 15 minutes, rinse again, then prepare and cook. This is one way to reduce the formation of acrylamide. Or boil for a few minutes, cool and freeze for future use. Another way is to cook potatoes with a fair amount of rosemary, which counteracts the acrylamide.

Solanine is a natural poison belonging to the potato to resist insects. Some people are more sensitive to it, especially those with gastrointestinal issues. The solanine content is most concentrated in the green coloration under the skin and in the eyes of the potato, and is accelerated when stored in the refrigerator. This can be eliminated or reduced by cutting out the eyes of the potatoes, by not consuming potatoes that have a green tinge under the skin, and storing them in a dark place.

For people who are diabetic, the potato is one food that should be avoided during their change to a better diet until blood sugar responses can be normalized.

3. Sweet Potatoes

Because it is a tuber, sweet potatoes have been put in the same category of other potatoes. Because of the high carotene content in sweet potatoes, they become a high anti-inflammatory, alkaline food. It does contain acrylamides just like any other tuber, but its high amount of the antioxidant Vitamin A may help in many ways. It is now viewed as one of the most nutritional foods in the human diet, and safe for diabetics.

4. Nuts

Warnings to not eat too many nuts are common in dietary recommendations, accused of contributing to weight gain, yet nuts are a highly nutritional natural food that make a great snack between meals, as long as they aren't coated in sugar, oils and unnatural coatings. Raw or roasted, they have omega 3 oil and vitamin E, magnesium, all good for heart health. Macadamia nuts have proven to lower LDL and triglyceride levels. Almonds benefit the heart and arteries with vitamin E, alkalize the body, and have a good amount of phosphorus to help with bone formation. Walnuts, with a high omega 3 content and very high anti-oxidant benefit, are great for the heart and ward off damage to cells. Keep them refrigerated when storing for a lengthy period of time to keep them from becoming rancid.

We are consuming more and more nut products lately, as the nut milks (almond, hazelnut, cashew) are becoming popular. Legumes of any kind interfere with absorption of certain needed nutrients such as iron and zinc, which makes supplementing with a quality multivitamin imperative.

5. Shellfish

Unless you are prone to gout, shellfish is highly beneficial to health. It is another food that has been shunned because of the cholesterol scare. Clams and scallops contain non-cholesterol sterols that actually decrease the absorption of cholesterol. Shellfish are low in fat, high in trace minerals and the antioxidant astaxanthin. Clams are high in vitamin B12. Shellfish are high in an easily digestible protein because of the lack of connective tissue as in most other animals.

6. Avocados

In the past, and still to some today, avocados have been shunned because of their high oil content, believing they would put on the pounds or contribute to heart disease. On the contrary, avocadoes improve vascular function. They are high in monounsaturated oil; this important type of fat assimilates easily for energy. They are good for the eyes and prostate, and a good source of glutathione, protein and Vitamin E.

7. Sardines

Sardines are not an attractive food, but they are full of omega 3 fats, high in selenium, and a good source of protein. Because they are at the bottom of the food chain, they are less likely to have notable levels of mercury or PCBs. They can be added to salads, and make a good option for including in hors d'oeuvres.

8. Coconut/Coconut Oil

For so very long, coconut has been on the no-no list because of its high saturated oil content, and scare of arterial blockage. It's now considered a superfood with huge healthful benefits with antiviral, antifungal and antibacterial effects. Its properties may improve wound healing and skin moisture, and is recognized as having anti-aging properties, and possible Alzheimer's prevention factors. This saturated fat does not easily oxidize or turn rancid, and is easily digested, keeping weight off and supplying energy. There are now healthful coconut product choices such as these: coconut flour, coconut oil, coconut sugar, coconut sugar nectar (similar to honey), coconut water, coconut milk, and of course the coconut flakes, dried or fresh.

Most Overrated Foods
- Milk
- Soy
- Agave
- Fruit juices

- Honey
- Egg Whites
- "Fat-Free", "Reduced Fat" commercial foods
- "Calcium Added" commercial foods
- "Sugar-Free" foods
- Vegan prepared foods
- Gluten-free prepared foods

1. Milk

Milk has been promoted for decades by the dairy industry as the most important beverage people can consume; here is why it is not:

Homogenization

Homogenization is done to keep the cream from separating from the liquid. This process infuses oxygen molecules into the fat cells in order for homogenization to occur, creating trans fat. This means that trans fat is being consumed, and this trans fat causes inflammation in the arteries. Homogenization has been described by Dr. Mercola, a raw milk advocate, as "a process that turns fat naturally present in the milk rancid and contributes to the formation of xanthine oxidase, a potentially damaging enzyme that has been shown to contribute to atherosclerosis." The homogenization process breaks up a certain enzyme in milk, which in this smaller state can then enter the bloodstream and react negatively against arterial walls.

The proteins inherent in raw milk are generally broken down easily during digestion. Homogenization disrupts this process, and allows these whole proteins to enter the bloodstream. These proteins are seen as foreign to the body and very often cause an allergic reaction, producing histamines, and then mucus. Homogenized milk proteins can sometime become triggers for autoimmune diseases such as rheumatoid arthritis or multiple sclerosis.

Pasteurization

Pasteurization converts milk proteins into mutated molecules that are foreign to the body when digested. Its purpose is to kill all bad bacteria in the milk. It also kills all the good bacteria, including enzymes. The main enzyme in milk is lactase. Lactase is there to digest the lactose in the milk. Without lactase within either the milk product or the body, humans become lactose intolerant. Lactose intolerance is yet another disorder caused by the disruptive processing of food. Phytase is also an important enzyme in milk because it helps the body digest the calcium. All enzymes are killed by pasteurization. Pasteurization also depletes nearly half the natural vitamins and minerals.

Calcium/Magnesium Ratio

The natural ratio of calcium and magnesium that a human should ingest, and does ingest if they were to eat a healthful natural diet of fruits and vegetables, is approximately 2:1. All fruits and vegetables naturally have content ratios of calcium and magnesium of around 2:1, some have 1:1, some 4:1; but on average they contain a ratio of 2:1. That is what the human body needs. Cow's milk is 11:1, meaning that the calcium intake far exceeds what the body needs to assimilate properly in the human body. This 11:1 ratio is designed for the nurturing of a calf to develop into a cow, not a human.

Allergy

Milk is one of the most allergic foods that humans consume, the most common food allergy in children; symptoms include wheezing, vomiting, hives and digestive problems. A milk allergy can create mucus and post-nasal drip.

Human Consumption

Humans are the only animals who consume milk after they are infants; and it is a milk that is not naturally made for humans.

Hormones

Cows are injected with artificially produced hormones in order to produce more milk. These hormones are passed on to the human who consumes the milk. Cow's milk has proven to be a contributor to prostate and breast cancer, likely because of these hormones, as well as the homogenization processing.

Grain Fed

Commercial cows are fed grains instead of grass that they were intended to eat. The effects of this passes on to us in the form of omega 6, causing the imbalance between omega 6 and omega 3 in our system.

Mammal Proteins

Mammals other than man contain the protein Neu5Gc. Humans have the Neu5Ac protein. When humans ingest the Neu5Gc in meats or milk, it is seen as an invasive germ and attacks it; this causes chronic inflammation. Neu5Gc is thus found in tumors in humans.

Cow Enzymes

Cow's milk contains an enzyme known as xanthine oxidase. When this enzyme is homogenized it inflames and damages arteries by producing superoxide radicals.

Casein Protein

Cow's milk contains 20 times more casein than human milk, making it very difficult to digest. Cow milk molecules are much larger than the human milk molecules that human babies ingest. Casein is a very allergenic protein, and has shown to contribute in some types of autoimmune disorders. Cow's milk proteins are strongly implicated in the development of Type 1 diabetes, as humans, especially infants, have trouble digesting this foreign protein in contrast to the human milk protein. As with any autoimmune disorder, the body becomes confused, and begins to attack particular organs, such as the pancreas.

Milk Proteins

Milk protein A1 and A2. A1 cows (mostly found in Europe, USA, Australia and New Zealand) have evolved from the A2 cows, creating a mutated protein which is not only an oxidant, but also triggers an autoimmune response in humans because it is identified by the body as a foreign invader. Studies have shown a reduction in autistic and schizophrenic symptoms with a decrease in A1 milk consumption. It is found to be an oxidant of LDL, contributing to arterial plaque. Whey protein is a concentration of milk proteins, and should be avoided along with all dairy products by anyone with any kind of health issue to rule out its effects.

Lactose Intolerance

As babies, the human is equipped with the lactase enzyme in order to sufficiently digest milk. As the human matures, the lactase enzyme is no longer produced naturally in the body. This is because the body knows that mother's milk for nurturing babies is no longer necessary. Therefore, the lactose in cow's milk and all dairy products cannot be sufficiently digested by humans because there is a lack of lactase enzymes to digest it properly (especially since the cow lactase enzyme in milk is destroyed in pasteurization). This is where "lactose intolerance" begins, creating discomfort in the stomach. This is not the same as a milk allergy.

Vitamin D

Vitamin D was added to milk in the early 20th century. Since milk had become a staple in the human diet, it was picked as the best method to get the minimum amount of Vitamin D in the human body in order to stop the epidemic of rickets that was occurring. The added amount of Vitamin D is 94 i.u. per 8 ounces. Vitamin D is not an inherent component of cow's milk, as most believe. The 94 units is sufficient in preventing rickets, however it is insignificant in the building of the human immune system, hormone maintenance, etc., which requires at least 1000 units per day, as recently reported.

Pregnancy and Milk

It is an old wives tale that pregnant women need to drink milk in order to breastfeed. Mother's milk does not come from cow's milk. Consuming cow's milk does not go directly intact to the breast. Mother's milk is made from nutrients in the complete diet of the mother; the more nutritious the foods, the more nutritious the milk. Drinking cow's milk has nothing to do with the production of human milk. Cow's milk is made for baby cows; human milk is made for baby humans.

If you wish to consume dairy, the safer dairy products to look for would be:

> European sourced dairy products
> Raw milk, yogurt or cheese
> Goat milk, yogurt or cheese
> Milk products produced from grass-fed cows or goats

If you decide to continue consuming dairy, here are two important tips for making it easier to assimilate in the body:

a. Take between 100 and 200mg. magnesium (citrate, aspartate, orotate, malate) right before indulging in any milk product – ice cream, glass of milk, cheese, yogurt, etc. This will make up for the low magnesium ratio related to the calcium contained in milk.

b. Take an enzyme tablet that contains lactase (there are also lactase drops available) right before eating any milk products. Adding it at the time of consumption will benefit digestion, and possibly avoid 'lactose intolerance'.

2. Soy

Soy has become one of the most pervasive ingredients in our diet lately, since its increase in popularity around 1970, and now is the largest export crop of the United States. It is used as a cow milk substitute, and very often as a food filler, especially in vegan products. However, there are two forms of soy available: organic fermented (highly nutritious) and non-fermented (highly processed). Fermented soy products include miso, tempeh, natto, edamame and soy sauce. These are the soy foods most popular in Asia. They are recognized as an anti-aging food. Tofu and soymilk can be found in fermented form (common in Asia), but the majority is unfermented. Basic soy contains a large amount of antinutrients that prevents vital nutrients from being absorbed in the body, yet fermenting soy destroys these components. In the making of soy protein concentrate, textured soy protein, hydrolyzed soy protein, and soy protein isolate, the proteins are processed in high heat and chemicals, resulting in toxic residue. Soy protein is most pervasive in vegan or vegetarian prepared foods. Because soy compounds resemble estrogen, it can have a hormonal effect on both males and females, including children. Men could have an overload of estrogen, and in using soy formula for babies, the same overload could occur, except with small bodies the effect could be extreme and harmful. An abundance of soy intake could interfere with thyroid function. Ninety percent of the soybean crop in America is genetically modified.

3. Agave

Agave has become a fad sweetener lately, mostly because of the industry's touting of it as not raising blood sugar levels. This is true, because of its high fructose content, and fructose keeps blood sugar tempered. The fructose is so high (70-90%) because of its processing procedure that it rivals high fructose corn syrup. High fructose is found to raise triglycerides, and is stored as body fat, leading to weight gain. Calorie content is the same as table sugar. It is highly inflammatory to the arteries, and has potential of causing liver problems. There is a distinct correlation between the start of the heightened consumption of HFCS in this country, and the rise in obesity, as it began to be added to sodas and then so many other foods. Agave consumption would be no different. The refining process for agave, because its starch and fiber are difficult to extract, involves various toxic chemicals, similar to those used for HFCS.

3. Fruit juices

Commercial fruit juices should be considered a refined food. They are, on the most part, stripped of all fiber and enzymes. With missing fiber, drinking fruit juice creates a blood sugar rush through the arteries, causing inflammation. Because commercial fruit juices must be pasteurized, the enzymes are eliminated. Juicing fruit at home will have the same effect, yet the enzymes will be in tact. There are some brands of fruit juice that actually contain added sugars, including high fructose corn syrup. Blending the whole fruit with water makes the best juice.

4. Honey

On the most part, honey is a healthful food, but its glorified traits belong to raw honey, not commercial honey. It is raw honey that holds the medicinal qualities; it's an anti-oxidant, it's anti-bacterial, and has lots of minerals, plus it assists in neutralizing free radical activity. Commercial honey is stripped of most of these benefits through processing and pasteurization. It has a high glycemic load while raw honey is lower. We now learn that many brands are not 100% honey. They have been adulterated with cheaper sugar substances; it may not even show on the ingredients, so be leery in your selections.

5. Egg Whites

Whole eggs were given a bad review decades ago, and so egg white products were developed for sale in markets and restaurants. But people have been missing out on the added benefits of the yolk in fear of cholesterol. Cholesterol in eggs is no longer the bad guy, and it is safe to say we can eat them. (See Eggs under "The Most Underrated Foods".) To me, eating just the egg whites is like eating a refined food, stripped of nutrients like choline and vitamin D; The yolk and egg white complement each other nutritionally, and eating both makes it a whole food, much like a whole grain. Their components work together for digestion and nutrient delivery.

6. "Fat-Free", "Reduced Fat" commercial foods

Over the past decades, people have been scared into eating foods low or free from fats, thinking fats or oils are either bad for health or will put on pounds. Fats are no longer the bad guy as they once were thought. Studies have shown that consuming less oils has been detrimental to our health; low-fat consumption has shown to do more harm than good. In addition, the so-called fat-free and reduced fat items have substituted sugars to make up in taste when fats are removed. We need fat in our diet. There are better fats or oils than others, however. I would suggest limiting the animal fats (dairy included), but the vegetable and nut oils recommended would be: coconut oil, flaxseed oil, and olive oil. Foods with healthy oils are: avocados, walnuts, cashews, wild salmon, and nut butters. Some people have been excluding these foods because of their high oil content, and now it's safe to say we all need them. These oils improve blood pressure, guard against arthritis and psoriasis, and improve skin texture (including rough heals), among many other things. So avoid foods that claim to be fat-free or reduced fat; these items are no longer warranted for a healthful diet. All oils are best unheated; olive oil and coconut oil are the safest to cook with.

7. "Calcium Added" commercial foods

The last decade brought about a calcium craze that swept through the media and food manufacturers, mostly because of the increase in cases of osteoporosis; but the reasons for this were incorrectly reported to the public; it is not the lack of calcium that is the problem. Reasons for bone deterioration has more to do with the increase in soda consumption, lack of magnesium in the diet, low estrogen in women and low testosterone in men, smoking, vitamin D deficiency, and lack of exercise. So many of these reasons are prevalent in our society lately. And when people believe that they need to replenish their calcium, an overload can occur, especially without the proper intake of magnesium or other minerals. Magnesium goes hand in hand with calcium, and it's imperative that it always accompanies an intake of calcium. Calcium needs magnesium and even vitamin D to assimilate properly within the body, otherwise the calcium will be misguided and calcium deposits will be created, two prominent places being in joints and arteries. Sodas are loaded with phosphoric acid, and this depletes calcium. Smoking will block the body from using calcium, vitamin D and estrogen properly. By adding more calcium to the body is adding to the problem. The other factors need to be addressed in order to stop the deterioration of bone. Therefore, avoid all commercial foods that say they have added calcium.

8. "Sugar-Free" foods

Sugar-free, no sugar added, sugarless foods are normally substituting refined sugar with chemically mutated refined sugar, such as sucralose or aspartame. These replacement additives are just as bad if not worse than white refined sugar. Always check the label ingredients; they could include maltodextrin, sorbitol, cornstarch as well; these are refined sugars related additives. Refer to the list of sugars included above in this chapter.

9. Vegan prepared foods

Foods that are prepared for vegan followers generally use a high amount of soy; but this soy is not the nutritious unfermented soy; these foods include the heavily processed forms of soy such as: soy protein concentrate, textured soy protein, and hydrolyzed soy protein. Soy protein isolate goes through an acid wash in aluminum tanks. Hydrolyzed proteins are processed with sulfuric acid and caustic soda.

These soy based meat alternative products for vegans are most often packed with artificial flavorings that include MSG that can give minor or major side effects; it can affect the brain, hormones, and nervous system.

There is a high chance that the soy in vegan products is genetically modified, since, according to the USDA, 94 percent of the US crop of soy in 2011 was genetically modified (GMO). Hydrolyzed corn protein is often used in vegan foods, and is also a GMO product. A high amount of wheat protein is generally used, which consists of a high amount of gluten. Anyone going vegan should seriously consider preparing more foods at home.

10. Gluten-free prepared foods

Gluten-free products have become fad lately, bought by not only those who have been diagnosed with celiac disease, but also many who feel they need to be eating gluten free to be healthier. These products may keep you void of gluten but aren't always healthful. Again, read the ingredients. Most of the time they are filled with ingredients void of nutrition, such as white rice, GMO corn flour and corn meal, and potato starch. Potato flour has the better nutritional content, as does brown rice when used in these products. Tapioca flour/starch is another common ingredient, and possesses minimal nutrients and no protein. Other flours, such as brown rice flour, quinoa, oats and sorghum, can be substituted in preparing home-cooked foods, rather than buying the readymade gluten-free products that are cheaply made, and less nutritious.

Research indicates that celiac disease may be prevented by breastfeeding and refraining from feeding babies any gluten grains for the first two years of life. For many, the intestinal lining has been compromised from ingesting toxins and refined foods over the years, and wheat gluten can exacerbate any intestinal problems, especially since it has also become a popular food additive. Gluten proteins are top food offenders, and we could all benefit by consuming less, but gluten-free prepared products are not the answer. Many who think they are gluten-intolerant and haven't been checked, should find out; find a certified nutritionist. Your issues may be something else.

Top Anti-Inflammatory Foods
- Peppers
- Wild Salmon
- Kelp

- Blueberries
- Walnuts
- Sardines
- Extra-virgin olive oil
- Cruciferous vegetables: Kale, broccoli, cauliflower, cabbage, brussel sprouts, bok choy
- Ginger
- Garlic

Top Antioxidant Foods

Starting with the highest score. Discrepancies in the order prevail throughout different reports, as with the oxygen radical absorbance capacity (ORAC) report, however these listed are undisputedly among the highest in antioxidant levels. Fruits in this list refer to whole foods and not juices.

- Raw Cacao Powder
- Legumes/Beans (Red, Kidney, Pinto, et al.)
- Berries
- Cranberries
- Artichokes
- Prunes
- Apples
- Pecans
- Cherries
- Russet Potatoes

These foods hold the keys to fighting wayward damaged cells within the body that can eventually mutate and reproduce abnormally. This is where antioxidants need to step in and destroy the wayward cell, or free radical. If we do not take in enough of these hero foods, then the damage continues into disease.

Top Supplements to Take Daily

Over the years we have learned that food alone is not enough to strengthen our immune system, live longer, and be our healthiest as we live longer. It's found that foods of today are lacking in nutrients because of deficient soils, and because of all the additives, chemicals, dyes and anti-nutrient foods such as trans fats, extra nutrients are needed to counteract their negative effects. Refined foods lack nutrients of all sorts, and are truly the main problem in the American diet.

Five categories of those who need to take supplements:

1. **Those who take pharmaceutical drugs**
   All drugs are toxic and require antioxidants to counterattack, and each drug depletes different vitamins and minerals from the body, for example, statins deplete COQ10.

2. **Anyone over 40**
   As we age, loss of vitamins/minerals is a natural occurrence.

3. **Anyone with a health issue**
   Disease clearly means that the immune system has been jeopardized, and is deficient in protection, making our body unequipped with the proper supportive natural nutrients such as antioxidants found in healthful fruits and vegetables.

4. **Anyone eating a diet of refined foods**
   Nutrients lost through refining, as well as the addition of chemical additives, warrants the need to replenish them.

5. **Those who choose to be proactive in health**
   Making sure the body is armed with an adequate supply of antioxidants, phytonutrients, and such helps keep illness at bay at any age.

Supplementation can be of benefit as long as the diet you choose to practice is the healthiest it can be. Without foods packed with nutrients, supplementing will not be able to carry the load of making you healthy. They should be used as complements. These supplements listed below are the least that should be taken to help keep a guard against disease.

Keep in mind that supplements are manmade, whether they say

natural or not. Someone had to process them to fit into a small pill. In my research, I am hard pressed to find a perfect multivitamin; perfect being one that includes 'natural' vitamin A (coming from a natural source), plus all the attributes listed below, but I did find one; it's quite expensive but has all the best features – liquid form, natural vitamin A, organic, comprehensive ingredients: IntraMax by DruckerLabs.

There is an overload of brands out there to choose from, and not all multivitamins are created equal. Most commercial products found in drug stores and department stores are of lesser quality, put together by pharmaceutical or smaller companies that merely want a piece of the retail market, using inferior ingredients to save money in costs and increase profit. Many multi-level supplement companies do the same, or the ingredients may be good, but the product overpriced. Ingredients should always be scrutinized.

Deciphering good ingredients from the inferior is very difficult for the common consumer. This is why I encourage everyone to purchase from a reputable health store. When the ingredients include such toxic additives as boric acid and dyes, then they should not be purchased. Also, purchasing a supplement because you think it might help may not be beneficial; again consult a nutritionist as to what supplements you may need for certain situations. Vitamins and minerals all work together in different ways, and purchasing just one singular supplement may be of no help, or may not even be the one that's really needed with your particular issue. It's a good idea to consult a nutritionist for recommendations on types and brands of supplements. Keep in mind that with any supplement, it's not just the type of vitamin, mineral or herb, that's important, it's the origin, it's form, or how it's made. This is discussed below.

The highest benefits we can obtain are through an abundance of natural healthful foods, while using supplementation as backup and enforcement.

Recommended multivitamins:
> *Source Naturals Life Force tablets (Green and original)*
> *Garden of Life Vitamin Code*
> *IntraMax (especially for complex health issues)*

Top Supplements ...*the basic minimum*

- Quality Multi-Vitamin/Mineral
- Probiotic
- Antioxidant
- Vitamin C (2 or 3 times a day)
- Omega 3 oil
- Vitamin D3
- **Magnesium (*especially for heart patients*)

1. Quality multi-vitamin/mineral

A quality multi-vitamin/mineral supplement is the basis for ensuring a healthful system. The quality of a good supplement depends on many different aspects of them. Any of these can be jeopardized in order to save money in production; check these before purchasing:

What forms of vitamins and minerals are included?

There are several forms of vitamins and minerals used in the composition of multiple supplements; some synthetic, some from natural sources. Three simple *red flags* to look for right away in a multiple are the following ingredients; these red flags will indicate if there was more consideration of quality and benefits than the saving of money expended on producing the product:

- **Cyanocobalamin;** should be methylcobalamin (the quality form of B12)
- **Magnesium Oxide** (the cheapest and least bioavailable; most commonly used, may do more harm than good); should be Magnesium Chloride, Chelate, Orotate, Citrate, or Gluconate. In fact, if the word **oxide** appears anywhere within the ingredients, avoid it.
- **Vitamin E** as **dl**-alpha (the synthetic form); should be d-alpha (the more natural form, having two times greater cellular activity)

These three ingredients should be checked immediately before purchasing to determine if this is an inferior multi-vitamin supplement.

If the manufacturer does not identify the particular forms of each nutrient, then this also is a red flag, and should be avoided. If the list only states Vitamin A, Vitamin D, Vitamin E, etc., without being accompanied by their proper name, then avoid it.

The quantity of each vitamin and mineral contained in the formula

The quantity of vitamins and minerals are expressed in milligrams (mg) micrograms (mcg), or international units (iu). In many supplements, the quantities will be lower, yielding less potency. Checking the quantities of the B vitamins is a good place to start.

- **B vitamin contents** (see B1) should show at least 5 mg., preferably over 10 mg, for each of the B complex vitamins

How many tablets or capsules are required to take each day to equal their indicated potency?

This can confuse many people. Two different supplements could indicate the same milligrams of certain ingredients, such as 10,000 mg. of beta carotene in each, yet if you look closely, one will require 2 or 3 tablets per day, while the other requires just one.

Check the pricing compared to how many supplements needed in a day; they may be overpriced for what you are getting. If one brand costs $10 for 100 capsules, and 2 a day equals the listed ingredients, and another costs $15 for 100 capsules, and 1 a day equals the same listed ingredients, then you can see that the $15 purchase is the better choice.

The number of different vitamins and minerals included

There are hundreds of nutrients that can be included in a multiple vitamin. Some may list 40, while another may only list 10. Part of the value comes down to how many good ingredients are included.

2. Probiotics

Our intestinal tract is supposed to be full of good bacteria to keep our immune system functioning properly, thus keeping us well. The gut is the basis of our immune system. With toxic foods, over-the-counter and prescription drugs and chemicals, the good bacteria are destroyed, and the bad bacteria begin to proliferate. Once the bad bacteria take over, disease has a good chance of beginning. Taking a quality probiotic supplement will ensure that the intestinal tract is armed with this good bacteria. Look for a supplement that contains several (at least 5) strains of bacteria; they will be listed on the label, such as L. rhamnosus, L.casei, B.lactis, L.acidophilus, B.longum, L. plantarum. Yogurt is touted as a good source of probiotic, but it's really not. Yogurts are usually full of sugar, and bad bacteria feed on sugar, so it is actually counterproductive. Yogurts are pasteurized, and it's difficult to find out if the product was pasteurized before or after the probiotics were included. Yogurts tend to have only one or two strains of bacteria. And lastly, yogurt is again a milk product, and not all people can digest and assimilate dairy properly. Choose a probiotic that needs refrigeration. Tests have shown that others are not as effective. Since probiotics are real live bugs, they should be contained as such, and kept cool and alive. Probiotics should always be taken during the time antibiotics are taken, in order to keep a large supply in the gut for the immune system. Just take them about 2 hours away from the drugs.

Recommended dosage is one supplement 1 or 2 times daily

3. Antioxidant

We all can use the help of a good anti-oxidant supplement as our food sources are tainted with chemicals, toxins and free radicals. Natural antioxidants are found in fruits and vegetables but we don't consume enough compared to the foods we eat that are anti-nutrient, such as over-cooked foods, trans fats and hydrogenated oils, and chemically-sourced food additives. My favorite antioxidant supplement is curcumin. Its realm of benefits cover cancer, gallbladder maintenance, hormone balance, digestion, joint function, helps the immune system and liver health. For other great antioxidants, see below - **Top Anti-Inflammatory and Anti-Oxidant Supplements.**

Recommended dosage is one supplement daily

4. Vitamin C

Vitamin C is much more than a supplement for colds and flu. It is one of the best vitamins for arterial health. Anyone concerned with blood pressure, plaque and heart disease should be taking it, as it helps with the elasticity of the arteries, and combats oxidative damage. It's not widely known that Vitamin C is an antioxidant. It is an adjunct to other antioxidants, giving them support in their effectiveness, especially Vitamin E. Since Vitamin C goes through the body quickly, targeting areas of need then released through urine, it is best to take it two or three times a day to constantly keep it in the system working for you.

Recommended dosage is 500-1000 mg., 2 or 3 times daily

5. Omega 3 oil

With the overabundance of Omega 6 oils in the American diet, we can all benefit by taking Omega 3 supplements to help balance these two important essential fatty acids. Our intake of omega 3 oils was much higher before our animal feeds were changed to grains. Most of our Omega 6 intake comes from either added oils in processed foods, oils used in frying at home or deep frying in restaurants. Omega 3 oils are found in seafood, grass-fed beef, walnuts, flaxseed, beans, spinach, and other various vegetables. Supplementing this nutrient helps with reducing inflammation, improves joint health, lowers triglycerides and elevates HDL.

Recommended dosage is EPA 400 mg., plus 300 DHA once or twice daily; both are found together in Omega 3 supplements

6. Vitamin D3

In our world of working long hours and having limited exposure to sunlight during winter months, staying indoors, and covering our bodies with layers of clothing, or the weeks and months of darkness brought by the winter solstice near the world poles, we need to supplement with Vitamin D. Winter depression in weather-filled cities like Seattle has been identified possibly as a deficiency of Vitamin D. The only true sources of this vitamin, other than sunlight, are fish, oysters, beef liver, egg yolks and mushrooms. Vitamin D deficiency affects the teeth, bones, arteries, blood pressure, brain health, depression and hormones. This is one nutrient that has been found to be lost in refined foods. The outbreak of rickets almost a century ago incited the government to have Vitamin D included in milk to alleviate the problem. But now we find the amount to stave off rickets is far too minor to aid the human body in achieving optimum health, one aspect being aiding in staving off cancer.

Recommended dosage is 2,000-5,000 iu daily

7. **Magnesium

Calcium has been played up as the hugely deficient mineral in our diets, when in fact it is most likely magnesium. Calcium and magnesium work together, therefore calcium should never be taken without magnesium, yet magnesium can be taken alone. Magnesium is the number one mineral to aid the heart muscle. Because so many have been supplementing with calcium without magnesium, arterial and heart problems can accelerate. Calcium deficiency is a usual reason given for bone loss, yet calcium cannot make bone unless there is magnesium; the intake of calcium may go into plaque or calcium deposits by not being directed by magnesium. Drinking soda in fact pulls calcium from bones. Far too much calcium is coming from dairy, which has been identified by many professionals to be an inadequate source. Magnesium helps regulate heart rhythm, blood pressure, and guards against kidney stones and constipation. It relaxes muscles and nerves. It is a highly necessary supplement since it is so often depleted in refined foods and deficient soils. This deficiency could very well be contributing to any current health problem.

Recommended dosage is 1 tsp 1-2 times daily in the powder form of
magnesium citrate or glycinate (necessary as well in any pill form of calcium)

Top Anti-Inflammatory and Antioxidant Supplements

- Alpha Lipoic Acid
- NAC

- Curcumin/Turmeric
- Vitamin C
- Fresh Garlic/Capsules
- Ginger

- Omega 3
- Ubiquinol/COQ10
- Astaxanthin

Other effective supplements:

- Selenium
- Vitamin A
- Green Tea
- Resveratrol
- Cayenne

- S.O.D.
- Pycnogenol
- Bromelain
- Ginkgo Biloba
- Vitamin E

Glutathione is the *Number One* anti-inflammatory/antioxidant that exists naturally within the body, and the most abundant, but diminishes with aging and with illness or stress of any kind. In fact, getting tested for glutathione levels can determine just how sick you may be. It is recommended that glutathione be replenished in times of major disease or stress to help the body help itself recover. There are glutathione supplements, however, taken orally in pill form they are not as potent as in its natural state, or may not even survive traveling the intestines at all. It can be injected into the body by a reputable doctor or at health clinics but this can be very expensive. There are two forms that may prove to be beneficial; one is a gel to rub into the skin over the liver, and the other a liquid form that is reported to be just as good as the injected form. It is called liposomal glutathione, uniquely mixed with phosphatidylcholine, and available on the web.

Glutathione can also be created internally by taking its catalyst antioxidants, either Alpha Lipoic Acid or N-Acetyl Cysteine (NAC). And it is also created by eating the foods that contain cysteine, glutamic acid and glycine: *meat, poultry, fish, eggs, dairy products, red peppers, garlic, onions, broccoli, Brussel sprouts, oats, and wheat germ.*

Consult a qualified nutritionist for the best supplement plan for your issues and situation.

"The best and most efficient pharmacy is within your own system"

~ Robert C. Peale

Chapter 7

Transitioning

Changes are very difficult things to confront in any realm of life. It is somewhat illogical to think that a person who has eaten a certain way, eaten certain foods throughout their life would suddenly be willing to eat the most extreme, healthiest diet. Even far too many of those who find they have suddenly contracted a serious or life-threatening disease cannot bring themselves to give up their foods of security – like a smoker who has smoked for thirty years. Who wants to give up everything they've enjoyed over twenty, thirty, fifty years of eating?

Transitioning is about becoming aware of the foods you eat, and about the choices you have in eating more healthfully. Transitioning is not about going from unhealthy eating to a totally raw, unconventional diet, and getting you to change completely overnight. It is about transitioning into eating better foods at a pace each person is comfortable with. As a person learns how our foods have been altered into unnatural substances that are detrimental rather than beneficial, the awakening may trigger more of a motivation to change their diets, and especially if that person contracts more and more ailments as they age.

Transitioning into a healthful daily diet takes time and vigilance. Most people are too busy, and their minds over indulged in other priorities to research and immerse themselves into the complexities of nutritional eating. This guide is meant to simplify your options in moving in the right direction concerning meals, supplements, and dietary habits with the goal of being healthier.

There are those who want others to think they eat right but don't; there are those who think they are eating right but aren't; there are those who want to believe they are eating right but fool themselves. Then there are those who don't even bother thinking about it; they just eat what they want with abandon.

9 out of 10 people will not self-administer natural medicine because of at least one of the following reasons:

1. Not believing that natural medicine/natural nutritional changes can make a difference or correct disorders, and think they are inferior to traditional medicine, albeit, drugs.

2. Apprehension of giving up comfort foods and regular eating habits.

3. Not wanting to make the effort and taking time it requires to research, self-administer and adhere to a natural health regimen.

4. Not having the understanding of what to do, how it works, and not having a nutritionist or proper authority to explain how it all works, instruct on what to do and what to get, especially since doctors generally do not offer nutritional advice. Feeling lost in an unfamiliar territory of health knowledge.

5. Wanting the easy fix of prescription drugs, having more familiarity to drugs rather than health foods and nutritional guidelines.

6. Reluctant to do anything unless their doctor says so. The doctor is the authority.

Beginning The Transition

The art of creating a nutritious lifestyle is time-consuming and commanding of our daily thought process, and it does in fact get in the way of our individual routines. This makes way to the easily accessible unhealthful menus at the majority of eating establishments, and the packaged, refined foods in all supermarkets. It comes down to whether we feel or understand that the inconvenience and effort are worth it.

The preparation involved in eating more healthful foods is unfortunately more time-consuming than anyone is used to; it's not an eat-and-run, friendly circumstance. There is a continual thought process involved in always being vigilant about what is the better choice in foods, more trips to the supermarket in order to maintain fresh foods, and more preparation time in cutting, mixing, cooking slowly, etc. These are big drawbacks to eating healthfully.

If you have a very busy daily schedule and want to begin a transition from unhealthful eating habits to anything better, you might want to consider doing this: whenever possible use disposable dishes and utensils to cut down on the time needed for cleanup. Using disposable dishes and utensils will be very helpful in keeping you from experiencing frenzy. Another thing is to plan meals for a week, and also cook several dishes at a time that can be eaten over several days.

So many books about nutritious eating have great factual, helpful information, yet tend to want to push people into changing from bad to perfect eating habits instantly, and a lot of the times they do not tell you the whys and hows of it all. Change should be at your own pace, while you better understand why the change is so important.

Part of the goal is to change your instinctive thinking about eating. That is, when you are about to make food choices, it will be in the front of your mind to determine what ingredients are contained in the foods you are about to order at the restaurant; when you are buying foods at the grocery store, you will read the ingredients on the labels; you will choose the fresh vegetables over the canned; when you think of getting popcorn at the movies, you will think about the high salt content and unhealthful, trans-fat oil they use, and have the willpower to resist buying it. These changes are commitment to transitioning to a healthful lifestyle.

There are basically four tiers of common diets:

Worst as we all know includes the "junk foods"; and there are some foods that people think are healthful but are not. It also encompasses the many ways of cooking, and preparation habits. These are foods that people who don't think about health when they eat them; these foods are eaten for hunger's sake.

Poor/Fair are usually those foods that people are tricked into believing are healthful, and some may have some good qualities. Without the proper knowledge people think they are eating something healthy, such as a margarine that touts that it contains the healthful substance of yogurt, yet also might contain hydrogenated oil. It includes foods that are easier to prepare.

Good refers to foods putting your body in the right direction, without negative effects; just short of the ultimate, optimum diet. It will definitely help keep you out of harms way.

Optimum contains all the proper foods and supplements, and ways of eating and cooking that are known at this particular point in time as the best you can give your body to be and stay healthy. One aspect of the optimum tier of eating healthy is eating more raw foods. Optimum, most importantly, eliminates all refined, packaged, processed foods, and includes only organic produce.

But who's to say what really is optimal, since so many different opinions are permeating our media, and information changes constantly over the years. We just have to keep moving in the right direction.

Chapter 8

Food Group Transitioning

Here are major food groups, showing the unhealthful to the OPTIMUM choices in each group. Use this chart for determining your desired choices for replacement or elimination of foods in your diet on your road to becoming healthier.

Note: The term 'free radicals' will be frequently used throughout this chapter. A free radical is a molecule that has been altered or damaged, losing an electron through interaction with oxygen molecules in a process called oxidation. The damage can occur through the breakdown of foods (usually processed foods the body sees as foreign matter) or through exposure to pollution, tobacco smoke, chemicals, etc. These free radicals are thus known as oxidants. Once they've lost an electron, they are on the prowl (free) to find that missing electron; one is then stolen from another molecule, and the chain reaction is begun. Free radicals are multiplied, cells are damaged, and disease sets in.

BACON

WORST   Pork bacon

Traditional bacon comes from pigs fed with GM corn and soy, and treated with additives; The main concern and a big negative is that bacon is enjoyed pan-fried at extremely high heat; Since bacon has a high amount of fat that is exposed to extremely high heat, this fat will become oxidized. Meats, especially bacon, pan-fried at high heats have been found to induce tumor growth, much like trans fat. Bacon also becomes oxidized when exposed to air for a shorter period of time than other meats. Highest of any animal in heterocyclic amines, a chemical formed through cooking that has been found to contribute to cancer. Another concern has been the nitrites used in curing, but is reported that many vegetables have more nitrites than bacon since the use of nitrites in curing has been overall reduced. Another concern with bacon is that it has a very high salt content. This amount covers a person's daily maximum allowance for salt.

Two interesting theories concerning pork: 1) It has been suggested that pigs do not have sweat glands, and therefore cannot sweat out the toxins in their bodies. Their huge layer of fat retains the higher-than-normal amount of toxins, also because there are no blood vessels connected to the fat that would help circulate the toxins within the system. Their quick digestive process does not give time to expel toxins. Pigs incubate viruses (flu), and carry parasites. These all have potential to remain in flesh, and be passed on to humans. 2) Religious groups contend that the bible and other documents declare that pigs are "unclean," and command that we should not even "touch their carcass" (*Leviticus 11:8*).

POOR/FAIR   Turkey bacon, Soy bacon

Turkey and soy bacon are processed, mechanically separated and formed into slabs, and cut into strips. Soy bacon may contain textured soy protein concentrate, wheat gluten, corn gluten, sugars, egg whites. Turkey bacon may contain corn syrup, sodium nitrite, sugar.

GOOD

100% grass-fed/pastured beef bacon (raised responsibly), uncured, naturally cured with no nitrites, sugars, additives; baked, broiled or low-temp, slow cooked.

Generally cut from slabs like regular bacon, has less fat, and fewer additives; some are made from grass-fed beef with no nitrites. Cooked slowly or baked, this form of bacon can give the beneficial nutrients of mammal meat without the added toxins.

OPTIMUM   *No bacon*

An unnecessary addition of saturated, and potentially oxidized animal fat or meat that forms free radicals harmful to cells.

BEVERAGES – *FRUIT JUICE*

WORST   *Sugared drinks, commercial fruit juices, pasteurized*

All canned, jarred, bottled, or carton fruit juices must be pasteurized by law, eliminating enzymes and killing GOOD bacteria. The added sugar in many juice drinks is unnecessary and highly toxic to the system by introducing higher amounts of fructose than what is already in fruit juice; there is no fiber in standard commercial fruit juices, allowing sugar to rush too fast through the body causing inflammation.

POOR/FAIR   *Whole-fruit juice (w/pulp, skin, etc.); freshly squeezed juices, Pasteurized*

Pasteurization kills all the GOOD bacteria within fruits and vegetables, whether it's made from whole fruit or not. Freshly squeezed still contains no fiber. Juices without the fiber and peel instantly inflame the arteries (inflammation), and cause an instant rise in blood sugar.

GOOD   *Whole-fruit juices (pulp, skin), unpasteurized*

Making juice in a blender with the skin and pulp slows down the assimilation of sugar within the body, delaying blood sugar increases, and avoiding blood sugar spikes. Fruit juice made by any method is still adding more unnecessary natural fructose to the body. Whole, unpasteurized fruit juice should still be limited to one a day at the most.

OPTIMUM   *No fruit juice; replace with water*

Depending on age, the body is made up of 45%-70% water and is the only liquid the body needs. Add natural lemon or lime juice for refreshing flavor; lime juice has the least amount of natural sugar of all fruits, then lemon. All other fruits have at least 5 times the sugar content.

BEVERAGES - *VEGETABLE JUICE*

WORST   *Commercial packaged vegetable juices, sugar added*

All canned, jarred, bottled, or carton vegetable juices must be pasteurized by law, eliminating enzymes and killing GOOD bacteria. The addition of sugar is unnecessarily adding the refined toxin to the system, adding to inflammation.

POOR/FAIR   *Commercial packaged vegetable juices without sugar*

These too are pasteurized. Elimination of added sugar is a plus.

GOOD   *Freshly squeezed vegetable juices*

Juicing the vegetables leaves out the peel and fiber necessary for intestinal, arterial health, but they have proven to have qualities of healing and cleansing the organs by delivering them easily through the system.

OPTIMUM   *Whole-vegetable juices (pulp, skin included),*
                     unpasteurized

Making juice with the skin and pulp gives high fiber and
phytonutrients, and delivers them quickly with little aid of
digestion.

BEVERAGES – MAMMAL MILK (COW/GOAT, etc.)

WORST   *Pasteurized/homogenized milk,*
                     sugared/flavored milk

There are a dozen reasons humans should not consume milk;
these are listed in Chapter 6 (Most Overrated Foods). Adding
sugars to milk products simply add fuel to the negativity.

POOR/FAIR   *Raw milk; unpasteurized kefir, organic*

If milk is preferred, then raw milk has far less negative aspects
than pasteurized/homogenized milk. Unpasteurized kefir tops
any milk beverage simply because it a fermented product.

GOOD   *Raw organic goat milk*

Goat's milk is preferred over cow milk because of its smaller fat
molecules for easier digestion, plus it is considered to be closer in
nutrient components than cow milk. More people throughout the
world consume more goat milk than milk from cows.

OPTIMUM   *Water, organic white tea (unsweetened); No*
                     dairy

Water is always the best choice, and most natural choice, for
quenching the thirst. Nothing more is necessary. White tea is the
next choice, and is the most nutritious tea, having the least
amount of fluoride. The nutritional value of milk has been

overstated by the dairy marketing campaign ever since the introduction of pasteurized commercial milk.

BEVERAGES – *ALTERNATIVE MILKS*

WORST   *Soy*

Soybeans contain the highest amount of phytates and enzyme inhibitors considered 'anti-nutrients'. These block the uptake of nutrients, and block natural enzyme activity. Soy is also a natural phytoestrogen food that can contribute to getting too much estrogen in the system, especially for men and children, and can disrupt thyroid.

POOR/FAIR   *Any alternative milk with sugars added*

Any drink with added sugars are counterproductive and adds to acidity. A negative to boxed milk alternatives are the added synthetic forms of vitamins.

GOOD   *Coconut, Almond, Hemp, Brown Rice, Oat Milk - without sugars added*

All of these are alkaline drinks, except brown rice milk is acidic. Alternative milks are still processed foods with additives, but they are not pasteurized or homogenized. They offer a good form of protein, minerals and fiber, more so than dairy. Carrageenan, a seaweed extract, is a common additive to alternative milks, and it does cause allergies in some people; if someone feels discomfort in the stomach or in sinuses after consuming a drink with carrageenan, then it's a sign of an allergy. Trying a homemade version would verify if the allergy exists. Cashew milk has yet to be commercialized.

OPTIMUM   *Homemade Cashew, Coconut, Almond, Hemp,*
Brown Rice, Oat Milk – without sugar

Freshly homemade milks of course do not go through commercial processing nor contain additives.

BEVERAGES – COMMERCIAL SODAS, ENERGY DRINKS, FLAVORED OR ENHANCED WATERS

WORST   *Any commercial soda (regular or diet), energy*
drink that contains some form of sugar

All soft drinks, energy drinks, and some water drinks are first and foremost sugar. Any drinks with added sugars are anti-nutritive, and adds to acidity. Most have caffeine, phosphoric acid, dyes and chemical sweeteners. Phosphoric acid, an ingredient found in commercial sodas, is linked to osteoporosis, kidney disease and kidney stones; it is a chemical commonly used as a rust remover.

POOR/FAIR   *'Natural' Flavored or Vitamin Waters*

Some natural flavored and so-called vitamin enriched waters do have sugar added or artificial sweeteners. Be on the look out for agave, sucralose and acesulfame potassium. Any small amount of vitamins included are negated by the sugars.

GOOD   *Sparkling, flavored water w/o sugar or*
sweetener

Carbonated water has not been found to harm bones or teeth. There are some sparkling waters that have a small amount of natural flavor, such as lemon or lime; these are acceptable. Those with too much added fruit juice, which is basically fructose, contribute more to your daily sugar allowance.

OPTIMUM *Low sodium mineral water, sparkling, plain or with natural lemon/lime juice*

International and domestic mineral waters add beneficial minerals to your diet missing from filtered tap water, and is void of chlorine and fluoride. All natural mineral waters are different, however; some contain high amounts of sodium (Vichy Springs, Calistoga, Crystal Geyser, Penafiel, Badoit, Gerolsteiner, Appollanaris), and some do not contain adequate amounts of magnesium in ratio to calcium (Perrier, Saratoga). Those with the best scores are: San Pellegrino, Evian, Rosbacher, Vichy Novelle, La Croix.

BEVERAGES – *WATER*

Research indicates that alkaline water can create problems besides helping, since its composition is unnatural. Eating alkaline is far better without the high cost.

WORST *Plastic Bottled Water, Distilled Water, Sparkling Water*

Most bottled waters are exposing us to toxins that leach from the plastic; the best type of bottled waters are in glass containers. When plastic bottles become heated, possibly from cleaning them, or in the sun too long, the leaching is accelerated. On top of it all, the number of plastic bottles being discarded currently is astounding, and overwhelming our dumps. Unfortunately only about 2% are recycled. Many bottled waters are either just common filtered tap water from various parts of the country, or reverse osmosis water, e.g., Dasani. Distilled water is good at certain times for mediating certain health problems, but not for ongoing consumption. Distilled water is acidic as its exposed to the air. Sparkling waters have carbon dioxide added for the fizz, making it more acidic; and they are without minerals. Microorganisms cannot live in carbonated water, however.

*(**Alkaline water**: There are reports, pro and con; some say alkaline water is unnatural and disrupts the body; others say more alkaline the better; it's your choice.)*

POOR/FAIR   *Reverse Osmosis Water*

Reverse osmosis is the only filtering system that deletes every contaminant, chlorine and fluoride, but unfortunately it leaves none of the good minerals intact, including trace minerals. In order to get health benefits that otherwise would have been in natural water, one could add a few drops of a quality trace mineral supplement to their water daily, plus a quality, full spectrum multivitamin/mineral supplement daily.

GOOD   *Filtered Tap Water, Club Soda*

Tap water in America is generally safe as the cities are mandated to treat the water, removing contaminants by adding chlorine. Fluoride is added in an attempt to guard against tooth decay, but the use of this toxic chemical is currently being disputed, citing many health side effects from it. Fluoride can affect the thyroid, cause bone damage, joint pain and cognitive development. For those who would like to lower their exposure to fluoride, avoid fluoride toothpaste, mouthwash, Teflon pans, and black and green tea which have high amounts of fluoride; white tea contains very little, and tastes just as good. Club soda has added minerals, as well as sodium bicarbonate, all of which add alkalinity to the water; this offsets the acidity of the carbonation. The carbonation does not allow harmful microorganisms to survive. A lemon-lime club soda can help a person get off the diet soda craving.

OPTIMUM   *Filtered tap water, Mineral Waters*

Currently, tap water in America that goes through a whole-house water filter system as well as a faucet or refrigerator filter is the better choice. Home filters generally filter out chlorine and bacteria, and up to 50% of the fluoride depending on the brand of filter, leaving minerals like calcium and magnesium necessary for the body. Most faucet filters do not filter fluoride. However, there are no filters available as yet (other than reverse osmosis) that will delete 100% of the fluoride from the water. Until they can remove fluoride from city water, it's suggested to stay away from the other fluoride products to decrease exposure. Mineral waters (in glass bottles) can offer a good amount of beneficial natural nutrients.

BREADS / GRAINS

WORST *White breads, refined/white flour crackers, pasta, bagels, muffins, etc.; breads containing fructose, sugars, hydrogenated oils, read labels)*

Most breads found in supermarkets contain refined grains, hydrogenated oils, and many different forms of sugar: fructose, refined sugar, high-fructose corn syrup, corn syrup, honey, molasses.

POOR/FAIR *Whole grain products, sourdough*

If the label states 'whole grain' (without the term '100%') then by law it can contain up to 49% refined flour. The typical commercial sourdough of today is cheaply made by cutting corners, and does not have all the benefits of traditional properly-made sourdough bread. If it doesn't taste like sourdough, then it most likely is not a true sourdough, and lacks nutrients it is supposed to possess.

GOOD *100% Whole grain products, true sourdough*

100% means no refined flour used; a 100% whole grain. Sourdough breads are preferred because they are fermented, and all fermented foods have benefits of improving digestion, contain microflora (probiotics), contain enzymes, offsets gluten, adds protein, have additional vitamins. A good sourdough made properly gives good bacteria to the gut, vitamin K, and nutrients are more bioavailable.

OPTIMUM   *Organic, sprouted grain products; 100%*
                flourless; alkaline or gluten-free grains. Or, no
                grains at all, as some professionals advocate.

Sprouted grains are the most natural form of grains, minimally processed, and retain the most vitamins and minerals. These are the sprouts at the beginning of the grain growing process. With the full, unprocessed grain, the insulin spike that's present in consuming a ground flour is avoided. Grains such as oat, quinoa, buckwheat, amaranth, brown rice, without additives and sugars; sourdough versions of any of these.

BREAKFAST CEREALS

WORST   *With refined sugar, fructose, corn syrup;*
                made with refined flours

95% of commercial cereals contain ground, refined grains and some form of refined, acidic sugar. These ingredients contribute to insulin spikes, high blood pressure, arterial damage.

POOR/FAIR   *100% whole grains only, w/evaporated cane*
                juice, brown rice syrup, or honey

These are mostly ground into flakes or shapes. The whole grain gives added fiber and nutrients, yet the ground flour travels through the arteries still too fast. Added acidic sugar again contributes to blood sugar spikes.

GOOD   *Complete 100% whole grains not ground to*
                flour (flourless), e.g., puffed brown rice, puffed
                millet, oatmeal; Unsweetened or with xylitol,
                stevia, erythritol

Grains must be whole and not formed into shapes. 100% grains are whole, and retain bran, germ; the whole grain cleans the arteries, travels the arteries slowly, keeping blood sugar stable. These sweeteners do not raise blood sugar; are alkaline, not acidic.

OPTIMUM *Organic, non-GMO, complete 100% whole grains not ground to flour (flourless), e.g., puffed brown rice, puffed millet, oatmeal; unsweetened; or no grains at all*

Many professionals advocate that grains be avoided completely; some say grains offer benefits to health. It would be best to keep them at a minimum. Cereal, first of all, should not be the staple of your breakfast; a good protein must be present. For optimum health, sugar should be avoided wherever and whenever possible. Best choices are whole grain, unprocessed, unrefined, in its original form.

CHEESE

WORST *Pasteurized cheese, processed cheese (American, etc.), cheese w/fillers (jarred)*

Cheese is a concentrated form of saturated fat and high in sodium. Pasteurized, homogenized dairy products (mammal fat) contribute to plaque build-up in the arteries and chronic inflammation. Processing and pasteurization add to inflammation and free radicals, and kills natural enzymes.

POOR/FAIR *Raw bovine (cow) cheese*

Raw cheese means it's made from the milk that comes directly from the cow, avoids the processing, pasteurization, additives, and retains the healthful enzymes such as lactase (for lactose) needed for digestion.

GOOD   *Raw goat cheese, Parmigiano-Reggiano (preferably Italian-made)*

The fat molecules in raw goat cheese are smaller and easier to digest in humans, are more similar to human. More people throughout the world eat goat cheese than cow cheese. Parmigiano-Reggiano has almost no lactose, (should have) no fillers, and the proteins have been broken down into peptones, peptides and free amino acids because of its lengthy aging process, making it easy to digest – 45 minutes as opposed to the usual 4 hours for bovine protein, which can cause distress and fermentation in the gut.

OPTIMUM   *No dairy products*

Some professionals believe dairy products are unnecessary to the human diet, and with most people, are not well tolerated, counterproductive to our health and should be avoided. Some believe it is a necessary part of the human diet; and some believe only raw milk should be consumed. It's a common fear that avoiding dairy would eliminate calcium from the diet, yet the best form of calcium can be obtained through fruits, vegetables, grains and other forms of protein. See Chapter 6 for the facts about the negative effects of dairy on the human body.

CHIPS

WORST   *Flavored Chips*

Here are just some of the unnatural ingredients that can be found in either the flavored potato or corn chips on the market: **Maltodextrin**, Cheddar Cheese (Cultured Milk, Salt, Enzymes) American Cheese (Cultured Milk, Salt, Enzymes) **Whey, Partially Hydrogenated Soybean and Cottonseed Oil**, Disodium Phosphate, Lactic Acid, Citric Acid, **Artificial Colors (Yellow 5, including Yellow 6, Yellow 6 Lake, Yellow 5 Lake, Red 40, Blue 1)** Cream, Swiss

Cheese (Cultured Milk, Salt, Enzymes) Colby Cheese (Cultured Milk, Salt Enzymes) Nonfat Milk, Butter (Cream Salt, Annatto) Parmesan Cheese (Cultured Milk, Salt, Enzymes) **Whey Protein Concentrate, Sugar**, Monterey Jack Cheese (Cultured Milk, Salt, Enzymes) Natural Artificial Flavors and Yeast Extract, **Monosodium Glutamate**, Sour Cream (Culture Cream, Nonfat Milk) Dextrose, Onion Powder, Tomato Powder, Molasses Powder**, Molasses, Brown Sugar**, Garlic Powder, Chili Powder, **Sodium Diacetate**, Spices, Paprika and Extractives of Paprika, Natural Smoke Flavor, Worcestershire Sauce Powder, **Disodium Inosinate, Disodium Guanylate**, Mono- and Diglycerides, Vinegar, **Hydrolyzed (Corn, Soy and Wheat) Proteins**, **Beef Stock, Corn Syrup, Autolyzed Yeast Extract, Cornstarch**, **Soy Bran**, Gum Arabic, Tamarind and Glycerol…*and this list is actually all from one product.*

POOR/FAIR   *Potato Chips, Tortilla Chips*

Chips are normally deep fried in the cheapest and most unhealthful oils, creating free radicals. Potatoes, as they are fried at high heat, produce a chemical called acrylamide that is associated with a high risk of cancer.   Corn does produce acrylamides but not as much as potatoes, and corn offers an extreme amount of omega 6 to the diet. Both come with a lot of salt.

GOOD   *Packaged organic Blue Tortilla, Sweet Potato Chips (or Fries)*

These are not deemed 'GOOD' nutrition by any means, but as a snack they are safer than what you normally get on the shelf, and would have to be unflavored. Blue corn has slightly more nutrients; organic is a plus. It's difficult finding baked sweet potato chips or fries that are only sweet potato without any additives.

OPTIMUM   *Baked Plantain Chips, Baked Sweet Potato Chips (or Fries)*

Homemade baked sweet potato chips or fries can be made with very little or oil; baked plantain chips (just plantain without additives) can be purchased at Trader Joe's and online. Baking chips does not subject them to deep frying in oil. Baking both sweet potatoes and plantains would have a lower incident of acrylamide formation.

COOKING FOODS

WORST   *Deep frying, high heat, Aluminum, Teflon pan on high heat*

Deep-fried foods contribute to heart disease because of the high-temp oils altering their molecules. High heat destroys nutrients, enzymes, and alters molecules in cooking oils and foods, creating free radicals. Teflon releases toxic gases linked to cancer at high temps that can be infused into foods. Aluminum from pans can absorb into foods during cooking.

POOR/FAIR   *Sauté foods; aluminum, Teflon pans on lowest heat*

Slow-fry foods will retain more nutrients; cooking in aluminum or Teflon on low heat reduces chances of toxins expelling from the pan to the food, but they still exist.

GOOD   *Steamed, low-temp sauté, stainless steel or 'green' pans*

Steaming foods and low-temp sautéing will retain even more nutrients; stainless steel pans are a safer surface for cooking. 'Green pans' or ceramic are the latest improvement in cookware; these do not emit any harmful toxins or minerals.

OPTIMUM   *Mostly raw foods; some steamed/low-temp sauté vegetables*

Raw foods retain all the beneficial enzymes, while there are a few vegetables that are worthy of light cooking, such as tomatoes, which actually increases its cancer-fighting ability found in lycopene. Cooking vegetables in a soup base or sauce that you intend to consume as well, as opposed to boiling in water, allows you to consume the released vitamins and minerals.

DESSERTS – (Made With...)

WORST   *With refined sugar, refined flours, hydrogenated oils, dairy*

Typical desserts are the ultimate in nutritional detriment. Ingredients are totally acidic, refined and toxic, void of nutritional value. They are working against the body, not for it.

POOR/FAIR   *With evaporated cane juice, honey, partly whole grain*

These are ingredients that can give desserts some nutritional value, but more acidic sugars than need be. Still has some refined flour.

GOOD   *With xylitol, erythritol, stevia, luo han, sucanat, coconut sugar, whole fruit, 100% whole unrefined grains/nuts (unprocessed); cold-pressed oils (virgin coconut oil, high-oleic sunflower oil).*

These sugars are alkaline; ingredients are very low processed; all of these add nutritional value to the dessert, and less negative effects.

OPTIMUM   *Fresh fruit with skin, raw nuts*

Fruit has the natural sweetness our bodies can best utilize. Raw nuts can go nicely with any fruit.

<u>EGGS</u> - Sources

By law, poultry and pigs cannot be given hormones.

WORST   *Caged Hens, Fed w/Animal Protein, Grain, Soy, Corn, Additives, Treated with Antimicrobials/Antibiotics*

Inexpensive eggs tend to come from poultry that are caged in overcrowded enclosures where disease can be an issue, therefore antibiotics are generally put into the feed to keep them from getting sick. Contained in lower quality chicken feed is animal protein consisting of various animal meats, bovine bone meal, poultry byproducts, feather meal and fish meal; not normal to the natural poultry diet. Grains, soy and corn are also added, also unnatural. Additives can consist of sweeteners, flavor enhancers, color, lubricants, and more; all things unnatural to poultry diet.

POOR/FAIR   *Cage Free. Fed w/Animal Protein and/or Grains*

Most are housed in large barns (as opposed to cages) and actually do not go outdoors. Quarters are more spacious than cages. Some producers allow them limited outdoor access, but most do not go outdoors. These can be fed an all vegetarian diet or with animal protein. Nesting space is included.

GOOD   *Free Range Chickens, Vegetarian Diet, Organic*

Free range allows the chickens outdoor access, but it is unknown how much time is really spent outdoors. Organic means that the feed has to come from organic sources; vegetarian diet means no animal protein is fed to the poultry; another plus, however, poultry are not vegetarians; they should eat worms, grubs, seeds, bugs and grass. On a vegetarian diet they can be consuming soy, corn and other grains that contribute to inflammation.

OPTIMUM   *'Pastured', Free Range, no Soy, Corn, Grains*

Poultry feed without grains, and especially soy, is an upcoming trend that is highly welcomed, and about time, but is extremely rare. Pastured on grassy outdoor areas is the optimum. Grains are unnecessary and uncommon to poultry diets. Eggs developed from animals that are free to roam in fields, raised on diets of worms, grubs, seeds, bugs and grass, without grains and without antibiotics are exactly what our bodies need, and hopefully more of these types of farms are being planned. Pastured is a term now being used, but still we are unsure of how much outdoor access they really get.

EGGS - Cooking

WORST   *Packaged, dehydrated, processed, irradiated, over-cooked, cooked on high heat*

Packaged, dehydrated, processed eggs are used often in restaurants; over-cooked eggs on high heat will chemically denature the egg protein and degrade the nutritive value. Irradiated eggs are often used by the restaurant industry to guard against customers becoming sick from errant bacteria, and potential lawsuits, but irradiation makes eggs, as well as other foods, deficient in vitamins, minerals and enzymes.

POOR/FAIR   *Omelettes, egg whites only, scrambled, cooked on both sides/over-easy*

Omelettes by their design are too often over cooked on the outside, causing them to 'brown', and create acrylamide. There are properties in both the yolk and the egg white that work together for OPTIMUM benefit. The 'whole' egg is a 'whole' food, and should be kept that way for its highest nutritional value. There are some who have allergies to certain components of the yolk such as phosphatidylcholine, or an allergy to either egg white or yolk protein.

GOOD   *Hard-boiled, low-heat sunny side up*

It's best not to allow the yolk to touch the surface of the hot pan; the higher the heat, the more chance of oxidizing the cholesterol in the egg yolk. It's not cholesterol that is a problem, it is oxidized cholesterol that inflames the arteries, leading to arterial damage.

OPTIMUM   *Poached, Soft-Boiled, Raw*

Poached and soft-boiled eggs do not expose the yolk to the heated surface of the pan. Many advocate eating eggs raw, which I too endorse because of their natural intact nutrients and enzymes, however most people are afraid to eat them because of the salmonella scare, and it's understandable. However, only sick chickens lay eggs contaminated with salmonella, so the more reputable the farm, the safer we can feel. (Also, the healthier the person, the less effect salmonella will have on that person.)

FISH

Most fish contain varied amounts of mercury. There are certain parts of the country as well as the world where fish accumulate more mercury and contaminants than other areas. Fish listed below may be well known for generally having high mercury levels. We just have to be cautious, and not consume large amounts of any fish, allowing mostly wild salmon, especially sockeye. When it comes to children, it's advised that fish in general should be even less consumed; this is because a child is so small in ratio to the toxin and mercury content of the fish. In fact, in some areas babies are born already with high mercury levels. It is a sorry state that we are to avoid an otherwise highly nutritious food source. The list below will therefore have to sidestep the mercury and toxin controversies and focus on the basic nutrition of fish themselves, consumed in small quantities. It also has come to light that at least 30% of commercial fish is mislabeled and is not what you think it is. Countrywide investigations have verified the fraud. And escolar tops the list of fish being substituted for tuna in as much as 70% of the cases found. Tilapia is often substituted for red snapper; farmed salmon is often substituted for wild salmon. All said, fish that we purchase and consume are suspect no matter where it originates. There are just too many varieties of fish to list; I have limited it to a small group of popular fish.

WORST   *Farm-raised Salmon and other farmed fish, escolar*

Farmed salmon is the complete opposite of wild salmon when it comes to nutrition. Farmed salmon, because of what it is fed, and because they are given antibiotics, dyes, and exposed to more toxins, they are considered bad for your health, contributing to inflammation in the body, while wild salmon is one of the most nutritious foods to eat. Farmed fish have a high omega 6 content, a low amount of fish oil, and therefore highly contributes to arterial inflammation. Consuming escolar can cause cramping, nausea, diarrhea.

POOR/FAIR   *Canned tuna, other canned fish (other than salmon), grouper, orange roughy, whitefish*

Canned fish have two risks involved; a risk of contaminants during packaging, and the toxic element BPA included in the lining of cans. The life span of groupers (40 years) and orange roughy (100 years) gives the possibility of these fish accumulating higher amounts of contaminants in their flesh than most fish over time. Food purveyors, restaurants may offer whitefish, but what are you really getting? There are so many different fish put into this category; the true whitefish is found in the Great Lakes, but these lakes are known as high pollution waters.

GOOD   *Canned salmon, troll or pole-caught albacore tuna, farmed oysters, white-flesh fish, lake whitefish*

Canned salmon will always contain wild salmon because farmed salmon does not hold up in the canning process; wild is the safest canned fish by the way it is processed. Canned or wild tuna labeled as troll or pole-caught indicates the fishing method has been eco-conscious. Farmed oysters are a healthy, safe seafood because they aren't fed; only absorb nutrients from the waters, and only flourish in clean environments. Wild oysters on the other hand are subjected to polluted waters. White-flesh fish and lake whitefish have a milder taste, and have all the benefits expected from fish.

OPTIMUM   *Wild, freshly caught or frozen salmon; mackerel, sardines, herring, anchovies, tuna, shellfish, shrimp, lobster, prawns, crayfish, freshwater fish, mollusks (live in shell): clams, mussels, scallops, oysters*

Wild salmon is the most nutritious choice, especially sockeye. Mackerel is a nutritious fish with low environmental contaminants and high in omega 3. Smaller fish – sardines, herring, anchovies – are richer in omega 3 than larger fish, highly anti-inflammatory, and because of their short life span, accumulate less contaminants. Freshwater fish, mollusks are high in protein, low in fat; clams are rich in iron, oysters rich in zinc.

FLOUR

WORST   *Refined white flour of any grain*

Refined grains are one of the top health offenders, contributing to arterial inflammation, diabetes, weight gain, and increased triglycerides and blood pressure. These have a lack of fiber, bran and germ, and beneficial vitamins and minerals.

POOR/FAIR   *Whole grain flour (not stated 100% whole grain flour)*

If the bread is not stated as 100%, then most likely it only contains 51% whole grain, and the rest refined flour, because legally that's all that is required when saying it is 'whole' grain.

GOOD   *100% whole grain flour*

When labeled 100% whole grain, it must be by law, and will be 100%. All the beneficial qualities of whole grain remain.

OPTIMUM   *No flour or grains, or 100% of the grains not ground down to a flour consistency, sprouted*

The less grinding of grains, the more utilization of high fiber traveling through the intestinal tract, and cleaning it out as it should be. 100% sprouted is the best choice in this regard; sprouted grains are those that have just begun to germinate through contact with moisture, exploding with all the beneficial nutrients of virgin grain.

FRUIT

WORST — *Canned or jarred, with added sugar*

Fruit is cooked, eliminating all enzymes, many nutrients; Added sugar is unnecessary, adding to the amount of detrimental refined sugar that enters the body on a daily basis, which poses health problems.

POOR/FAIR — *Fruit, canned or jarred, with no added sugar*

Fruit is cooked, eliminating all enzymes, many nutrients; cans may expose the fruit to the toxin BPA that is in the lining of most cans.

GOOD — *Fresh or frozen fruits only, with or without peel*

Frozen fruit is just as nutritious as fresh fruit, and possibly more so, depending on how old the fresh fruit is. The longer it's been since the picking of fruit, the more nutrients have been lost.

OPTIMUM — *Organic fresh or frozen fruits only, with peel predominantly*

The skin on fruit is highly nutritious, and sometimes even more than the inner fruit itself, as it is with watermelon. Eating predominantly fruit that the skin can be eaten as well is the best choice, such as berries, cherries, apples.

FRUIT JUICES

WORST — *Fruit Juices with added sugar, bottled, jarred, Packaged Juices*

All packaged juices have been pasteurized, which eliminates

natural enzymes, and there is most likely no fiber left with the juice. Fruit is already full of fructose, and adding yet unnatural sugar contributes to high blood sugar and potential health problems.

POOR/FAIR   *Fruit Juices without added sugar, bottled, jarred, packaged Juices*

Plain fruit juice commercially packaged have been pasteurized, no enzymes, no fiber. The juice is left to race through the arteries causing inflammation because of the lack of fiber.

GOOD   *Juiced or blended whole raw fruits, fresh or frozen*

Plain raw, whole fruits retain the enzymes and fiber.

OPTIMUM   *No juices; replace with water; fresh/frozen fruits eaten whole only*

It's best to limit the consumption of fruit to lower our consumption of fructose.

HAMBURGERS

WORST   *Typical hamburgers, meatless/veggie burgers*

The worst part of the typical hamburger is the bun; generally made with refined flour, hydrogenated oils, sugars; many contain high fructose corn syrup and azodicarbonamide, a toxic dough conditioner; the meat is from grain-fed cows, again adding more omega 6 to the body. The bun contributes to diabetes, and both contribute to arterial damage. Meatless burgers generally contain soy protein concentrate, textured soy flour (both highly processed products), and sugar and/or high fructose corn syrup.

POOR/FAIR   *Grain-fed beef with 100% whole-wheat buns*

The 100% whole-wheat bun will give added nutrients, but generally they will most likely still be filled with sugars, hydrogenated oils and additives; the grain-fed beef contributes more omega 6 to the body.

GOOD   *Grass-fed beef, 100% whole-wheat bun w/o additives*

Grass-fed beef will contribute more omega 3 oils to the body, and the 100% whole-wheat bun gives added nutrients, especially w/o any added sugars, hydrogenated oils, additives.

OPTIMUM   *Grass-fed beef, turkey or chicken patty, 100% sprouted grain bun, no sugars/hydrogenated oil, no nitrites, Sunshine brand burgers*

A sprouted grain bun (w/o additives) is the best choice since it is mostly unrefined. Commercial turkey or chicken patties are mostly unadulterated meats; Weight Watchers getting a star for having no negative additives. Sunshine brand burgers are another good commercial patty made with brown rice and without additives.

HOT DOGS

***Sodium nitrates come from vegetables such as celery; celery is very often used as the source for using in the curing process for meats. During this process, the sodium **nitrate** turns into sodium **nitrite**. It is claimed that as the sodium nitrite is cooked, it becomes a toxic element. Some manufacturers claim that since vegetables contain sodium nitrate, and digestion converts it to sodium nitrite, then there is no difference between that and what is contained in the cured meats; however, the difference is that the conversion that has already taken place in the cured meat, and then exposed to high heats, thus converts it to a toxic element. The sodium*

nitrite that is converted within the stomach is converted naturally, and is not exposed to high heat.

Here are the differences: One is natural in fresh foods, and one is chemically synthesized. The vegetable sodium nitrite is converted to nitrate in the body naturally; the cured-meat nitrite is artificially converted to nitrate in the processing of the meat. The vegetable containing the nitrate, also contains antioxidants that counteract the effect of any nitrate conversion in the body. Plus Vitamin C helps diminish the ill effect, which is also present in most of these vegetables. This is where I believe the difference between safe and toxic lies. Best to take a vitamin C and an antioxidant food or supplement when eating processed meats.

WORST   *All commercial, typical hot dogs, pork/beef; additives; refined bun*

Typically all commercial hot dogs contain sodium nitrite, a chemical that may cause migraines, and when cooked, the high heat boosts the formation of cancer-causing elements. The buns are full of refined flour, hydrogenated oils, sugars; most contain high fructose corn syrup and azodicarbonamide, a toxic dough conditioner;

POOR/FAIR *Beef, turkey, chicken; whole grain bun*

Here we still have meats that will contain sugars and nitrates; the whole grain bun is still not 100% whole grain (most likely 51%), and could contain the sugars, hydrogenated oils, additives, etc.

GOOD   *Grass-fed beef, turkey/chicken non-grain/ corn/soy fed, 100% whole grain bun, no sugars/hydrogenated oil/additives*

Grass-fed meats, no additive, no hormone meats are the best; a 100% whole grain bun without the additives mentioned gives the proper fiber content.

OPTIMUM   *Organic, grass-fed beef, turkey/chicken, 100% sprouted grain bun, no sugars/hydrogenated oil/additives in either the bun or hot dog.*

Organic meats are a plus; and sprouted grain buns are the most nutritious. I recommend a brand called AppleGate or the equivalent; their products are mostly grass-fed (check the label), no nitrates, no sugars. Two brands - Food for Life and Alvarado St. – make nutritious buns without sugars and additives.

KETCHUP/CATSUP

WORST   *Commercial, typical ketchup*

Typical ingredients in common ketchup include: high fructose corn syrup and/or corn syrup, white distilled vinegar.

POOR/FAIR   *Organic ketchup*

Most likely the ingredients are the same, but they are organic products, including organic white sugar.

GOOD   *Homemade ketchup made with fresh tomatoes, xylitol, sucanat, apple cider vinegar*

These ingredients are far more healthful, and make the condiment an alkaline food rather than acidic.

OPTIMUM   *No ketchup; fresh, organic tomatoes to flavor food*

Because we need not add more sugar substances to our bodies, it's best to not feel we need to add ketchup to our food. Adding tomatoes in some form is the better choice.

MARGARINE/SPREADS

WORST   *Hydrogenated margarines; pasteurized butter*

The common, standard margarines in a stick form are most likely hydrogenated (molecular structure altered); this is done to keep it solid in a stick. Made from vegetable oils, they are filled with preservatives and artificial flavorings; some contain whey, which most people don't realize, and if you are trying to avoid dairy, you're not. Sticks of regular butter are basically made with cream; they do list 'natural flavorings' also as an ingredient, but it's never revealed what these 'natural flavorings' are. Butter manufacturers now whip their butters, and sell them in tubs, and generally contain the same ingredients...cream and natural flavorings. But all butters are pasteurized and homogenized, making them an unhealthful processed food.

POOR/FAIR   *Non-hydrogenated spreads (tub, soft margarines, e.g.), Raw butter*

There are now margarines sold in tubs that are more spreadable, healthier than the original stick margarines, but beware, there are only a few that are somewhat healthier: Melt, Earth Balance Coconut Spread, Earth Balance Soy-Free. Remember all oils are still processed foods. Raw butter, without additives, is not pasteurized or homogenized.

GOOD   *Oil/liquid form only – virgin/cold/expeller-pressed: Olive oil, coconut oil, flaxseed oil, sunflower, palm kernel, Homemade margarine, Raw organic butter*

If an oil spread is needed, then try just the liquid oil itself; a homemade margarine beats all commercial spreads (find a GOOD recipe in the recipe section of this book); there would be no preservatives or artificial flavorings or additives. Raw organic butter is the best choice when wanting to use a true butter; all natural nutrients are intact, without having hormones, steroids, antibiotics, etc.

OPTIMUM   *None*

All oils are processed foods, all being a part of a whole food at the time of extraction. We are inundated with oils in our diet, and eliminating as much as possible, and eating the food from which it came would be better for our health. If you are looking for an oily spread, try natural nut butters or avocado, which are full of natural oils.

MAMMAL MEATS

WORST   *Deep-fried, over-cooked mammal meats, grain-fed/corn-fed*

The combination of deep frying and mammal meats can be deadly, literally; high heat, grilling, deep frying all contribute to the potential of acrylamides forming in the meat, as well as any food, which can contribute to cancer. By consuming grains or corn, which is not the natural diet of mammals (bovine, pig, lamb, bison, etc.), the animals have more health problems and therefore require antibiotics that are passed on through the meat; the grains themselves are passed on through the meat, which contributes more omega 6 to our already over-consumption of omega 6 as related to omega 3 that are more beneficial; a grass-fed animal will contribute more of the beneficial omega 3 to our diet. Plus, by eating grains, animals are more susceptible to E. coli growth in their stomachs from the acidic nature of grains.

POOR/FAIR   *Ground meats: beef, bison, etc.*

Prepackaged ground meats are more susceptible to bacteria from handling and machinery. There is a substance called 'pink slime' that is being added to ground beef reportedly in close to 70% of grocery meat departments. These are scrapings from the bones, including muscle connective tissue, that are sprayed with ammonium hydroxide to kill potential E. coli and salmonella, used as an inexpensive filler.

GOOD   *Fed on grass, organic, no hormones,*
                 home-ground

Animals have historically been raised grazing in grass fields. Then came the money-saving diets of grain and corn. Now, more and more animals are being raised on grass once again because it's found to produce a much healthier finished meat for humans, and we are beginning to ask for it. It's becoming more and more possible to find grass-fed meat, organic without hormones and antibiotics. Grinding it to hamburger at home is a trustworthy decision, knowing that there is no chance of contamination or additives.

OPTIMUM   *Grass-fed, no hormones; Raw, steamed, boiled*

Steamed and boiled meat do not sound appetizing, but this is a way to avoid acrylamides that form when meats are cooked at high heat on hot surfaces, creating the 'browning' effect. Broiling can cut down on the acrylamides, but the cooking would need to stop before the 'browning' occurred. Eating raw meats, as with all foods, is usually the most healthful, as long as the source is perfectly sanitary, the beef is organic, grass-fed, and void of chemicals, hormones, etc. This is hard to find in modern day food supplies. Boiled meats can be in the form of soups and stews. Raw meats contain all the necessary enzymes to digest the meat, and by cooking they are destroyed. Our bodies are actually fully equipped to handle raw meat. Raw meats are consumed and enjoyed in many countries like Japan, France, Germany, Ethiopia, and Korea. But mainly it's Americans who have a problem eating raw meat. We eat Steak Tartare and many have their steak rare;

we find no problem in eating raw fish in sushi or Ahi tuna; and cooking beef has proven to not keep us from harmful bacteria as we do have salmonella or e. coli outbreaks at hamburger outlets or restaurants occasionally; even raw vegetables can become contaminated. (Mammal meat consumption should be cut in half.)

MAYONNAISE

WORST
Commercial salad dressing/mayonnaise w/sugar, white vinegar, hydrogenated oil, soybean oil

There are no commercial mayonnaise or salad dressings that compare to the nutritional benefits of homemade. They are all pasteurized, lacking enzymes, many vitamins and minerals; most contain sugar, white vinegar, and low quality oils.

POOR/FAIR
Commercial mayonnaise w/apple cider vinegar, no sugar (e.g., Trader Joe's yellow label mayonnaise)

The only mayonnaise I have found that does not contain sugar, uses apple cider vinegar, and is an expeller pressed oil is Trader Joe's yellow label mayonnaise.

GOOD
Homemade mayonnaise (see recipe chapter)

By making homemade mayonnaise, you benefit by the enzymes found in the ingredients; no pasteurization, no sugar. Use raw, unfiltered apple cider vinegar, organic expeller pressed oil such as olive, sunflower or coconut, and raw egg, all nutritious.

OPTIMUM
None

Using mayonnaise merely adds to your daily consumption of processed oils. The less oils consumed daily, the better.

MILK *(see BEVERAGES)*

NUTS

All raw and roasted nuts, legumes, seeds and grains naturally contain enzyme inhibitors (phytic acid, tannins, goitrogens). Nature put them there to keep them from germinating too soon. But these enzyme inhibitors also inhibit healthful actions in the body, such as digestion, natural enzymes that control inflammation, and they inhibit many vitamins from being absorbed.

WORST   *Peanuts: Honey-roasted, sugared, Dry Roasted, using hydrogenated oils*

Peanuts are the most unhealthful 'nut' to consume; first of all, it is not a nut; it is what is called a legume, belonging to the same family as the dry beans (kidney, soy, pinto, lentils, etc.). Legumes, including peanuts, are an inflammatory food, and the peanut protein is unfortunately highly allergenic, one of the most common of allergy causing foods. Dry roasted have gained a reputation as being healthier than regular peanuts because they are prepared without oil, but this is another case of misinterpretation of nutritional facts of our food. Dry roasting may not add oil for roasting, and can be more healthful because of this, but here are typical ingredients that most manufacturers add to their dry roasted peanuts: monosodium glutamate, cornstarch, sugar, corn syrup solids, hydrolyzed soy protein, maltodextrin, and other additives. Honey roasted nuts could commonly include all or some of these ingredients: fructose, cornstarch, sugar, corn syrup, potato starch, partially hydrogenated soybean oil, and more. Peanuts roasted in oil, are just that…peanuts, and oil, salted or unsalted; roasted would be the better choice. Make sure hydrogenated oils are not used.

POOR/FAIR   *Roasted Nuts, Dry Roasted Nuts, Salted*

Roasting or drying does diminish some nutrients. Dry roasted nuts of any kind are most likely to have the same unhealthful added ingredients as the dry-roasted peanuts (usually not macadamia nuts). Always read the ingredients on labels. Nuts sold as roasted in oil, generally have no other ingredients, but check just in case. Nuts roasted in oil can go rancid easier than raw, but all nuts with their high content of oil can still go rancid. All nuts should be kept in the refrigerator. The abundance of salt found in processed salted nuts is something to consider and try to avoid.

GOOD   *Raw Nuts, Dry Roasted Macadamia*

Raw nuts are without additives, as are most dry roasted macadamia nuts; they contain higher amounts of natural nutrients, fiber and protein. They do, however, still have enzyme inhibitors that suppress the enzymes needed for digestion. Almonds, by law, are pasteurized, so they actually are not raw.

OPTIMUM   *Sprouted, then dried*

Sprouted nuts (all legumes, grains, seeds) are becoming more available, as well as do-it-yourself sprouting at home, as their nutritional value is made known. Sprouting nuts is a time-consuming process, but it's the best way to eat nuts; it's possibly what Mother Nature had intended. Nuts are protected by enzyme inhibitors until they fall to the ground and become moistened by rain or morning dew. Then the sprouting of the nut begins over several days. When they sprout, the toxic inhibitors are released, the natural enzymes for proper digestion become available, and the nutrients become more readily bioavailable. At home, nuts can be put through the entire sprouting process or soaked for a few hours and rinsed to release much of these toxic inhibitors, then dried and stored.

OILS FOR COOKING FOODS – *(never deep fry ANY foods)*

*Since you **WILL NO LONGER** deep fry foods in oil, there is no need to focus on what is called the 'high flash point' or 'high smoke point', meaning looking for oils that don't 'smoke' when they reach high temperatures, because once the smoking begins, the toxins and free radicals are released. These oils that can reach high heat without smoking are generally more refined, and are generally more unhealthful. So either way you lose healthwise. Destruction of omega 3 oils when cooked can lead to free radicals.*

WORST　　　　*Trans Fats, Hydrogenated Oils, Flaxseed Oil*

There is a controversy among professionals about the formation of trans fat in high heat cooking, but basically both trans fats and hydrogenated oils have been altered. Hydrogenated oil has been developed in order to have food products stay on the shelves longer, to make margarine harden like butter, and to be able to use deep-frying oils longer before turning rancid. These oils are processed using unsaturated oils, and not saturated. In essence, it is an attempt to mimic saturated oil, as saturated oil was deemed the villain decades ago. Instead, they are so altered and processed that they create havoc and inflammation in the body, leading to heart disease, high blood pressure and cancer. Flaxseed, a highly nutritious oil, has the most amount of omega 3 of any oil, and for this reason it should never be used in cooking foods.

POOR/FAIR　　　*Grapeseed, Safflower, Corn, Cottonseed, Soybean, Peanut, Canola, Sesame Oil*

These oils, no matter how they are processed, are the highest in omega 6 content, and can highly contribute to inflammation in the body. Canola does have a GOOD amount of omega 3 and because of it, its omega 6 content tends to not promote inflammation, however, this oil is from a seed that was first 'bred' to be safe, then genetically modified to be tolerant to herbicides. It is also one oil that uses hexane in its processing; soybean is another.

GOOD *Virgin/Cold-Pressed/Expeller-Pressed Coconut, Palm, Olive, Avocado, Macadamia Oil*

Oils extracted using these methods are the only oils to buy. This means minimal processing, only from the first pressing of the food. The more processing of an oil, the more refined it becomes, and the more unhealthful. High heat in processing causes mutated fatty acids. The best cooking oils because of their low omega 3, and lower omega 6 content, but have high nutritional value, include: avocado, coconut, olive, almond, macadamia, palm.

OPTIMUM *No Oils, Whole Foods*

All oils are processed, and the most healthful way to obtain needed oils is through eating whole foods such as avocados, fish, nuts, seeds, coconuts, etc. It's never mandatory to use oils in cooking; they can be substituted with things such as coconut milk, applesauce and water. Heating or cooking oils always gives chance to altering their nutritional value even more so than what has been done by extracting it from the whole source.

OILS FOR NON-COOKED FOODS

WORST *Hydrogenated Oils, Processed Vegetable Oils*

These types of oils do not belong in any diet. The more processed the oil, the more havoc and inflammation are created in the body, leading to heart disease, high blood pressure and cancer.

POOR/FAIR *Safflower, Soy, Corn, Peanut, Sesame, Canola*

These types of oils have far too high of omega 6 content; this creates inflammation as well.

GOOD *Virgin/Cold-Pressed/Expeller-Pressed Coconut, Olive Oil, Flaxseed, Sunflower, Avocado, Macadamia, Almond*

These types of oil extraction allow minimal processing; the less processing, the less chance the body is subjected to free radicals. These types of oils are alkaline forming oils, with the least chance of inflammation.

OPTIMUM *No Oils, Whole Foods*

All oils are processed, and the most healthful way to obtain needed oils is through eating whole foods such as avocados, fish, nuts, seeds, coconuts, etc. Making dressings out of whipped avocado, chickpea, tahini, or almond butter is utilizing the whole food, and not just the oil.

PASTA

WORST *Standard, white refined flour pasta*

Refined flour pasta has been a staple for centuries in most countries, including Italy. It has all the beneficial fiber and nutrients taken out by removing the bran and germ of the grain. This contributes to diabetes, high blood sugar and inflammation.

POOR/FAIR *Whole grain pasta*

When the pasta is labeled as 'whole grain' it can be legally, and most likely is 49% refined flour. This is better than all of it refined, but still lacking a lot of nutrients. This form is a GOOD transition from refined to 100% grain pasta.

GOOD *100% whole grain pasta – 100% brown rice pasta*

Pasta labeled as 100% whole grain will be 100% whole grain and no refined flour is allowed. Once you get used to eating this pasta, you won't want to eat refined.

OPTIMUM *100% Sprouted Organic Grain Pasta (or no grains at all)*

Sprouted grain pasta gives you the best of the nutrients that come from sprouted grains; the enzyme inhibitors are gone and the enzymes for digestion are available. However, sprouted grain pasta requires getting used to; it has a very different texture.

Because of the growing amount of people with digestive problems including gluten intolerance, and the proliferation of manipulated grains, it is recommended by many professionals to avoid grains in the diet altogether.

PEANUT BUTTER

WORST *Contains Hydrogenated oils, sugar*

Common, everyday peanut butter as we know it is full of anti-nutrient ingredients. They could include high-fructose corn syrup, refined sugar, cornstarch, and hydrogenated oils. Ingredients must be read.

POOR/FAIR   *Powdered Peanut Butter*

This is not a real, whole food; essential oils are extracted, including vitamin E, rendering it a refined food; they usually contain added sugar.

GOOD   *All natural; mix half natural peanut butter/half almond butter (or cashew or macadamia)*

All natural requires stirring the oil in, but worth it; keeps solid in the refrigerator. Should contain only peanuts and salt (check ingredients). Since peanuts are highly inflammatory and acidic, and almonds are very alkaline, a GOOD practice is to mix half of each in a jar. This ends up tasting like peanut butter, and some people cannot acquire a taste for the almond butter in order to make the substitution. With the combination, the alkaline will downplay the acid, the added benefits of the almonds are a plus.

OPTIMUM   *No Peanut Butter; Instead Use Almond, Macadamia or Cashew, Sprouted Nut Butters*

It's best to consume less peanuts and more alkaline nuts such as almonds, macadamia and cashew. The butters made with these nuts are simply blended whole nuts; these contain only the nuts and possibly some salt. Sprouted nut butters are becoming available, which are even better, as they are easily digested.

POTATOES

Potatoes, when cooked properly, offer an abundance of nutrients. Our bodies thrive on starch, as it turns to glucose and energy. But to someone eating unhealthfully, or who has diabetes, potatoes should be avoided until their body is balanced, healthy, and free of diabetes.

WORST   *Deep-fried (French fries, Potato Chips, etc.),*
                      high heat surface, green, raw

High heat, especially deep frying, will bring out the toxic chemical acrylamide residing in potatoes. Deep fried potatoes are full of free radicals, and will cause an inflammatory effect within the body. Green or sprouted potatoes are exceptionally high in natural protective toxins, rendering them in the body. Potatoes are not easily digested when raw.

POOR/FAIR   *Eaten without skin, fresh or frozen, sautéed,*
                      Grilled, Broiled

Eating potatoes without the skin will cause a spike in blood sugar; the peel is the added fiber needed to slow the glycemic load on the arteries. Browning potatoes during sautéing, grilling and any high heat exposure, will release added potential cancer-causing toxins into the body when eaten.

GOOD   *Eaten with skin, baked, added in soups, boiling*

Potato skins offer exceptional fiber, an added amount of minerals and vitamins: iron, vitamin B, C, B6, copper, calcium, niacin and more. Potatoes added in soups or just boiled avoid any browning, and avoids acrylamides. Baking in casseroles, sauces in covered pans or foil will keep potatoes from browning, but baked potatoes are still subject to the formation of acrylamides.

OPTIMUM   *Organic, with skin; baked, broiled or boiled*
                      then chilled, Red Skinned, Purple

Potatoes can be a nutritious part of a healthful diet if they are prepared properly. Potatoes should not be eaten raw because of certain natural toxins; potatoes cannot be cooked on high heat surfaces because of certain natural toxins. However, as they are cooked at low temperatures, boiled, and soaked in water, and even chilled after cooking and before eating, they hold a load of vitamins and minerals. Tubers (such as potatoes) are eaten by a variety of cultures throughout the world as an integral part of healthful diets; treated with respect during preparation, they offer high vitamin C, high fiber, high potassium; always leaving the skin on, they are beneficial for the heart and blood pressure. When cooked then chilled (as in potato salad), their glycemic load is much lower than when eating them right after they've been cooked. Red skinned as well as the purple potatoes possess an added benefit of a nutrient called anthocyanin; this is what makes the foods of color become red, blue or purple. It helps protect against oxidative damage, may help eyesight, and may be an aid in cancer.

POULTRY

By law, poultry and pigs cannot be given hormones.

WORST *Caged, Fed w/Animal Protein, Grain, Soy, Corn, Additives; Treated with Antimicrobials/Antibiotics*

Poultry that are caged in overcrowded enclosures where disease can be an issue, generally have antibiotics put into the feed to keep them from getting sick. Contained in lower quality chicken feed is animal protein consisting of various animal meats, bovine bone meal, poultry byproducts, feather meal and fish meal; not normal to the natural poultry diet. Grains, soy and corn are also added, also unnatural. Additives in the feed can consist of sweeteners, flavor enhancers, color, lubricants, and more; all things unnatural to poultry diet.

POOR/FAIR *Cage Free. Fed w/Animal Protein and/or Grains*

There is controversy as to how often the so-called 'cage-free' chickens are allowed to roam outdoors on open land. These are either fed an all vegetarian diet or with animal protein.

GOOD   *Free Range Organic Chickens, Vegetarian Diet*

It may sound GOOD that poultry have been fed a vegetarian diet, but poultry are not vegetarians; nor do they wish to eat grains like soy and corn. Organic is a plus; vegetarian diet means no animal protein is fed to the poultry; another plus, however, poultry are not vegetarians; they should eat worms, grubs, seeds, bugs and grass. On a vegetarian diet they can be consuming soy, corn and other grains that contribute to inflammation.

OPTIMUM   *Free Range Organic, Fed Without Soy, Corn, Grains; Fed Worms, Grubs, Seeds, Grass*

Poultry feed without grains, and especially soy, is an upcoming trend that is highly welcomed, and about time. Grains are ingredients that are not necessary or common to the poultry animals' diets. A diet of the natural insects, seeds and grass found as they roam outdoors is the best.

RICE

WORST   *Instant White Rice, White Rice*

It's found that there is no difference in nutrient content between instant white rice and regular white rice. They both are lacking in fiber, vitamin E, choline, and others. They are high inflammatory, and cause blood sugar to rise quickly.

POOR/FAIR   *Brown Rice*

Brown rice has some added nutrients, and because it retains the bran and germ of the grain, the rise of blood sugar is much slower than white rice. Brown rice is more tolerable to diabetics. Studies show that those who eat brown rice have lower cholesterol.

GOOD   *Organic Brown Rice*

Organic eliminates hazardous chemical exposure.

OPTIMUM   *Organic Black Rice, Red Rice, Wild Rice*

These forms of rice contain added nutrients that brown rice does not possess, which are anthocyanins. This nutrient is also found in blueberries, and is a reason for blueberries to be touted as so nutritious; however, the rice is looked at as more beneficial because it does not have the fructose content that blueberries do. These are proving to be an excellent food in fighting cancer. It has been reported that they may be anti-inflammatory, beneficial in treating diabetes and ulcers. It is the dark, red, purple pigment properties of these foods of color that possess these anthocyanins. Wild rice has more protein, less inflammatory effect, more omega 3, more vitamin A, and a slower rise of blood sugar.

SALAD DRESSING

WORST   *Commercial, Restaurant, Ranch Dressings*

There may be a few healthful commercial salad dressings out there, but they are hard to find. Always read the labels. Most have sugars, inflammatory oils, hydrogenated oils, artificial colors, white vinegar, and monosodium glutamate. In fact, most of the popular ranch dressings contain all of these ingredients. The most popular ranch dressing on the market and in restaurants is the most requested because it contains a fair amount of monosodium glutamate. It appeals to the taste buds, and sets the craving to come back for more. It is never really known what is in restaurant dressings because we do not get to see labels and ingredients; it can be assumed that it is laden with sugar and cheaper oils. Most patrons think nothing of what is in the dressing, but for a health conscious person, speaking up for replacements can be an option; one option is to request olive oil and balsamic vinegar and lemon juice for your dressing. Hopefully they will not substitute the olive oil with a lesser quality oil, but we have no control. Another option is to bring your own dressing in a small travel container.

POOR/FAIR   *Homemade salad dressings made with ready-made dressing consisting of: Trader Joe's Yellow Label mayonnaise*

A quick way to make a homemade dressing is with a ready-made mayonnaise. The only worthwhile commercial mayonnaise I've found (on the west coast) is Trader Joe's with the yellow label. It can be used as a base for Thousand Island, curry, etc. These can be found in the recipe section.

GOOD   *Homemade dressings made with homemade mayonnaise, lemon juice, apple cider vinegar, balsamic vinegar, expeller-pressed oil, spices*

Any homemade dressing or homemade mayonnaise is by far more healthful than any commercial brand. Anywhere, we are hard-pressed to find a decent, healthful salad dressing without soy oil, canola oil, sugar, agave, white vinegar, etc. Using a homemade mayonnaise as a base, it's easy to concoct a tasty flavorful salad dressing. Or get creative with different ingredients, spices.

OPTIMUM   *Organic Ingredients, Lemon juice, apple cider vinegar, balsamic vinegar, expeller-pressed oil, spices*

Salad dressings are just a means to palette the dry greens going down the throat; another way to make something taste sweet to satisfy the sweet tooth. These are the best basic ingredients for any salad dressing, keeping the oil to less than 50%, and adding spices, fruits, garlic, seeds, etc., to make it your own.

SUGAR/SWEETENERS

WORST   *White sugar, fructose sweeteners, artificial sweeteners, agave*

Most people know that white sugar is a highly refined no-no. Most do not realize that artificial sweeteners such as Equal, Splenda, and the like (sucralose, aspartame), are counter-nutritious. The fact that they are chemically altered substances may contribute to diseases including cancer. Fructose as a sugar is highly inflammatory; as a sweetener, is it unnatural, being stripped of the fruit fiber that naturally comes with it. Using fructose as a sweetener may cause health problems involving the liver, heart and kidneys. GOOD marketing has made agave a respected sweetener, however, the truth is that its content is high fructose, causes inflammation, and is a highly refined product making it acidic.

POOR/FAIR   *Brown rice syrup, honey, turbinado*

The processing of these forms of sweetener cause them to be somewhat acidic, and they may tend to cause the blood sugar to spike.

GOOD   *Sucanat, Xylitol, Stevia, Raw Honey, Coconut Sugar, Maple Syrup, Molasses, Luo Han*

These forms of sugar or sweetener are closest to natural, and all are alkaline. Sucanat is the true brown sugar; it is made from the first pressing of the sugar cane juice with the natural molasses intact. Xylitol is natural from the birch tree, with a very low glycemic load. (Another form of xylitol is made from corn, but inferior.) Stevia is extracted from the stevia plant, and can be 300 times sweeter than sugar, and does not spike blood sugar, but does have an aftertaste. Raw honey spikes less than regular honey, and has more beneficial qualities. Coconut sugar also has a low glycemic load. Maple syrup has a high concentration of minerals, and less of a sugar spike than honey. Molasses is very similar to maple syrup in composition and benefits. Luo Han comes from monk fruit, is another low glycemic-load sweetener, and highly concentrated like stevia. It is difficult to find a true Luo Han that is not mixed with other sweeteners.

OPTIMUM　　　*No sugar products of any kind added to food, basic fruit*

It would not be the optimum thing to suggest a sweetener, and have it become overused, thus exposing an overload of glucose to someone's system. True sweeteners should be basic; down to the real whole fruit, allowing the fruit fiber to work with the juice to control any glucose surge. Our taste buds and bodies truly have been overexposed to too much over-refined, acidic, and chemically altered sugar throughout our lives. Even though a sugar is an alkaline, low glycemic load, and has beneficial nutrients, it is still a sugar, and will contribute to an individual's glucose intake, possibly causing an imbalance and overload of sugar.

SOY PRODUCTS

Most of the U.S. soy crop is genetically modified, commercially it is highly refined possibly with the use of toxic chemicals (hexane), and leads to hormonal imbalances and even miscarriages. All beans and grains contain natural protectants like phytates that can inhibit certain minerals from being absorbed by the body; soy happens to have much more than other beans, and the hull is harder to break down, meaning more processing. Soy also produces estrogenic isoflavones that can contribute estrogen to the body (especially harmful to males and children if consuming too much), and contains goitrogens that prove to slow thyroid function. On the other hand, soy contains high protein, has shown to lower triglycerides and LDL, and raise HDL. It can contribute estrogen when a woman is deficient, however can inhibit the production of testosterone in men. Asians have never included as much soy into their diets as the Americans now do. This is because we consume more processed soy, as they consume mostly the more natural, fermented soy products mentioned below. Processed soy has infiltrated our packaged foods, vegan foods, baked goods and more, much like refined sugar. Keeping our consumption down, and consuming more of the highly nutritious forms of soy would be worthwhile.

WORST   *Textured Soy, Vegetable Protein*

These are not the nutritious soy foods that the Asian culture has eaten over the centuries. For those who choose to follow a vegan diet, very much of the commercial, prepared foods offered are filled with textured soy protein because it's the simplest inexpensive answer to substituting for meat protein, but it is highly processed, very allergenic (one of the top eight), often containing monosodium glutamate (MSG). Some people may not eat mammal meat simply because it's mammal eating mammal, but at least it's a natural source of protein; textured soy protein is not; oil is removed, it's then soaked, heated or boiled, extruded into shapes, dried by ovens, then rehydrated. This is not a type of protein that seems safe to consume in high quantities. Better to be safe than sorry, and avoid consuming soy protein products.

POOR/FAIR   *Soy Milk, Soy Protein Isolate*

Soy milk has been promoted as a healthful replacement of cow's milk, but it actually does not have any added value, and is just as negative as milk in its own ways. Soy milk is heated to extremely high temperatures which destroys its natural component of cysteine (an aid to the immune system), and degenerates the soy protein, making it difficult to digest, and may cause intestinal discomforts.

GOOD   *Edamame*

Edamame is the immature soybean pod, are boiled in salty water, and can be served as a snack. It's a more natural way to obtain the soy protein.

OPTIMUM   *Tempeh, Natto, Miso, Soy Sauce,*
Fermented Soy Products

Fermented soy products are the type of soy foods that the Asian cultures have eaten for thousands of years. They understood the negatives of the soybean in the diet, and somehow thought to use the fermentation process to make it better. Fermentation, a healthful process that breaks down carbohydrates into simpler components, leaves the beneficial soy phytochemicals that promote health intact. Tempeh is nutty tasting, has a nougat-like texture in a cake form, and used in a variety of Asian dishes. Miso is a soybean paste full of minerals and fiber, added to soups and a variety of Asian dishes. Natto, fermented soybeans, contain a high amount of Vitamin K.

SOY SAUCE

WORST   *Soy Sauce with added salt, wheat, and caramel*

Soy sauce is a fermented soy condiment that has been used for centuries, but some American manufacturers have added caramel to appease palettes even more. Caramel is a sugar-based substance, and is unnatural and unnecessary in a soy sauce. Wheat or grain has been a base substance for the fermentation process of soy sauce, but it can be avoided, especially for gluten intolerance. Salt is a common ingredient in soy sauce, but more salt is often added; this can be avoided as well.

POOR/FAIR   *Soy Sauce, without caramel*

Look for soy sauce without caramel; you must read the ingredients carefully.

GOOD   *Soy Sauce, reduced salt, no caramel*

Look for soy sauce without caramel, with reduced salt; it will often say on the front label that it has in fact reduced salt, but you must also read the ingredients carefully to look for caramel.

OPTIMUM   *Soy Sauce, reduced salt, no wheat, no caramel*

This would be the best choice for soy sauce: low salt, gluten-free, and sugar free. San-J Organic (with the silver label) is one brand that accomplishes this.

TOMATOES

WORST   *Canned w/sugar, salt, stewed*

Never buy stewed tomatoes because they contain unnecessary sugar. Any vegetable in cans has potential toxic BPA contamination, but acidic foods, such as tomatoes causes it to leech out into the foods more readily.

POOR/FAIR   *Canned without sugar, low/no salt*

Eliminating the sugar content and lowering the salt content is a step in the right direction. Canned tomatoes most often contain citric acid in the ingredients as well. This is a small additional contribution to the acidic factor.

GOOD   *Jarred, without sugar, low/no salt*

Purchasing tomatoes in jars eliminates the potential of BPA leaching into the product.

OPTIMUM   *Fresh, organic*

Fresh organic tomatoes are always the best choice.

TORTILLAS

WORST   *White, refined flour tortillas; deep fried*

White refined flour tortillas are nothing but an anti-nutrient product; have little fiber, very few vitamins and minerals, most often hydrogenated oil (usually soy), and many chemical additives. Being a refined product, they are high inflammatory, and will spike the blood sugar. When you fry them, they may contribute free radicals, and higher inflammation.

POOR/FAIR   *Corn Tortillas, Whole Wheat Tortillas*

Corn tortillas generally do not have as many additives as flour tortillas, and the way that masa is prepared, it renders the corn a healthier choice than flour tortillas. Whole wheat tortillas of course offer more nutrients because of whole grain used, except it is only 51% whole grain; the other 49% could be refined white flour. They still most often contain a high amount of additives.

GOOD   *Organic 100% whole wheat or corn, w/no hydrogenated oil, no sugar*

100% whole wheat and corn are the better choices, both containing all of the grain, nothing refined. Make sure the flour tortillas do not have hydrogenated oils or sugar, or too many chemical additives.

OPTIMUM   *100% Brown Rice, Sprouted Grain*

100% brown rice tortillas are delicious, nutritious, and gluten-free; sprouted grain tortillas of course are highly nutritious compared to any other, but the texture has some getting used to.

VEGETABLES

WORST   Canned, Boiled

Keep away from as many canned foods, especially vegetables and fruit, as possible. They are exposed to BPA toxin, and are cooked at high heat, eradicating enzymes and most nutrients. Boiling vegetables will do the same (except in making soups, where the liquid is also consumed).

POOR/FAIR   Jarred Vegetables; Peeled Vegetables

Jarred vegetables avoid the toxin BPA, but the vegetables are still void of enzymes and most nutrients. Peeling vegetables eliminates a high amount of very beneficial fiber and added nutrients.

GOOD   Raw or Cooked at Low-Heat, Saute, Fresh or Frozen w/Peel

Cooking vegetables slowly with little liquid or oil will keep the loss of nutrients to a minimum. Raw is best with most vegetables; some can have a little added benefit if they are actually cooked, such as tomatoes. Both fresh and frozen vegetables are equally nutritious; always leave the peel intact for added nutrients and fiber.

OPTIMUM   Fresh or Frozen Organic Vegetables, Mostly Raw

Always choose organic when possible; raw vegetable consumption should be at least 50%.

VINEGAR

WORST   *White vinegar, white rice vinegar, balsamic (with sugar/caramel)*

White distilled vinegar is mostly made from grains, and is a high acidic food; the same with white rice vinegar. Most marinated foods contain distilled vinegar; I suggest rinsing of as much vinegar as possible for eating. The true balsamic vinegar does not contain caramel, a sugar additive. Use the white distilled vinegar for cleaning; that's its best usefulness.

POOR/FAIR   *Red wine vinegar, brown rice vinegar, Malt Vinegar; Balsamic (without sugar/caramel)*

Red wine vinegar and brown rice vinegar are from less refined sources, and are not as acidic. Balsamic vinegar without the caramel added is a much better choice, and close to neutral in pH.

GOOD   *Apple Cider Vinegar*

Apple cider vinegar comes from the alkaline fruit, and is an alkaline vinegar. It has many health benefits, especially for neutralizing the intestinal tract. It can be substituted in cooking any time vinegar is needed.

OPTIMUM   *Organic, Unrefined Apple Cider Vinegar w/'Mother' (mass of live nutrients & bacteria)*

The unrefined apple cider vinegar will have sediment at the bottom of the bottle. It has the yeast and fermentation by-products used in the fermentation process, and is of added benefit. Shake the bottle before pouring to include it in each use. This type of vinegar has numerous health benefits because of its highly alkaline nature. It may help in eradicating aches and pains, reduce blood pressure, help in digestion, GOOD for skin conditions, and weight loss. Its taste is potent, but it is, after all, medicinal.

YOGURT

Yogurt has claims of exceptional health benefits all around the world. In reality, the only difference between plain milk and yogurt is the beneficial bacteria called probiotics. Americans have chosen to turn yogurt, a possibly GOOD thing, into a dessert. By adding sugar, it becomes more palatable, and of course more marketable. But it has actually negated what yogurt is all about...the GOOD bacteria. Sugar feeds BAD bacteria, and therefore increases their numbers while decreasing the number of GOOD bacteria. Dairy is the number one cause of allergies, and sixty percent of humans are lactose intolerant.

WORST *Sweetened w/Sugar, Artificial Sweeteners, Fructose; Frozen Yogurt, Soy*

Today's yogurts are filled with refined sugars, artificial sweeteners, fructose, and even fillers. Some brands do not even ferment their yogurts long enough to have the bacteria proliferate enough to become truly thick, as normal yogurt should; instead they thicken the yogurt with cornstarch, food starch, gelatin, milk solids. This is the case with non-fat yogurt and soy yogurt as well, since they do not thicken as easily as whole-milk yogurt. Pectin is the best natural thickener that could be included. Dyes may also be included in the fruit flavored yogurts to help them look more colorful and appealing. There is nothing nutritional about frozen yogurt as well; it is loaded with even more sugar and additives.

POOR/FAIR *Unsweetened Goat or Cow, Greek style*

Yogurt, whether cow or goat, should be plainly milk and/or cream with bacteria, that's it. Greek style yogurt is when the whey is completely removed from yogurt; this is done to make it naturally as thick as can be. Whey is full of amino acids, so for those looking for nutrients, keeping the whey in yogurt is beneficial.

GOOD   *Organic Goat, Plain, Unsweetened, Grass-Fed*

Goat milk products are consumed far more throughout the world than cow milk products. Goat milk is actually closer in molecular makeup to human milk than cow. The most nutritious yogurt would be organic, grass-fed goat, without any sweeteners or additives.

OPTIMUM   *No Yogurt, No Dairy*

We are the only mammal that drinks milk from another mammal, and the only mammal that drinks milk after infancy. I profess that any dairy works mostly against our human system, and is unnecessary, citing that it can produce health problems that may never be realized; disorders may be medically determined to be caused by some other source, and never actually be resolved.

"Some people die at 25 and aren't buried until 75"

~ Benjamin Franklin

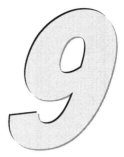

Chapter 9

Food Health-Factor Reference Chart

These charts are guidelines for eating the right foods in regard to your bodily concerns, and to make sure you maintain above a 60-40 pH ratio for the correct alkaline-acid balance.

The optimum ratio is 80% alkaline and 20% acid. The alkaline-acid range should not fall below 60% alkaline and 40% acid, or disease will have an easy road into the body.

The charts consist of the following Food Groups:

- Fruit
- Vegetables
- Meats/Fish
- Grain Foods/Flours
- Nuts/Seeds
- Eggs/Cheese/Dairy
- Beans/Legumes
- Oils/Fats
- Beverages
- Condiments
- Herbs/Spices
- Sweeteners

The *Health Factor Reference Chart* points out the various attributes of everyday foods that may trigger certain maladies. Please use it as a quick reference in planning your daily menus to avoid over-consumption of foods that may put you in harms way, or those that have already put you there.

Acid vs. Alkaline

There is a pH balance the body naturally maintains within our cells, tissues, fluids and organs to keep us alive. Mainstream medicine continues to disregard this balance as relevant to good health, yet its importance has become essential in the field of nutrition. It is verified that with trauma, such as major surgery, comes metabolic acidosis – a flooding of acidic components within the system, as the alkaline components such as magnesium and oxygen are depleted. It is known that the lack of oxygen impairs the cells, and believed that such disease as cancer then thrives in a low oxygen state; and the opposite is believed, that a high oxygen state will arrest the growth of diseased cells. The key to good health is making sure our diets contain a higher intake of alkaline foods than acidic foods; close to at least 60% alkaline and 40% acid. The current average diet is far below 50-50.

Of course, the body does work continually to bring back a balance pH in the system, but if acidic foods are continually fed into the body, then the body is overwhelmed, overworked, and cells have little chance to heal. Acidic foods tend to be meats, grains, legumes, processed foods. Alkaline foods tend to be fruits and vegetables.

Inflammatory vs. Anti-Inflammatory

Inflammation is the number one detriment to our arteries and health. Processed foods top the list of inflammatory foods. Although there are many fruits that are listed as inflammatory, don't let it scare you. The inflammatory rating pertains to the natural sugar content; this is a rating of inflammation that I feel is somewhat distorted. Whole fruits are full of so much fiber that counteracts the inflammation process, and these fruits contain natural compounds and phytochemicals that are known for anti-inflammatory effects in the body, such as cyanin, quercetin, and hesperidin; so fruit should not be pushed aside, except for certain fruits if you are diabetic. However, if inflammation is a problem in your system, eliminate any suspicious food, fruit or otherwise, to try to pinpoint the problem.

In one way, our bodies create a form of inflammation to fight off germs or repair an injury. This is the redness seen around a wound, or the fever that comes with the flu. The body is attacking the disruptive foreign bodies that made their way past the immune system. This type is helpful. The other form of inflammation comes from ingesting foods that the body identifies as foreign intruders and attacks. These foreign intruders are the foods that Mother Nature did not intend us to eat, like deep-fried potatoes or candy bars. The more we bombard our system with these types of foods, the harder the fight, the more injury to the arteries and cells. Most fruits, vegetables and herbs have natural healing components that are deemed 'anti-inflammatory' because they fight foreign, inflammatory invaders such as toxins and free radicals.

High Glycemic – Not for diabetics

The glycemic load is a rating system for foods that shows how fast and strong they can affect blood sugar. You will notice that most of the fruits marked as 'high glycemic' are fruits that are normally eaten without the skin. The skin is what can keep the blood sugar from spiking. As long as fruits are eaten with the skin, they can be a highly nutritious part of the diet. If you want to eat the skin of the papaya or banana, go right ahead; you can only benefit by its added fiber and nutritional value. The diabetic is best to avoid fruit that is not eaten with the skin or peel.

May Cause Allergies

These foods are more likely than others to contribute to allergic reactions in some people.

High Purines – Adds to gout

Most foods contain some amount of a natural compound called purines. When purines are broken down in the body, they form uric acid. A certain amount of uric acid is helpful to the body because it can serve as an antioxidant, but when high levels are continually introduced to the body, they tend to crystallize and accumulate in joints and tissue pockets (especially with a low intake of water) and thus creates the debilitating condition known as gout.

Inflames Arthritis

Most often, inflammatory arthritis is caused by eating an abundance of inflammatory foods; mainly processed, acidic foods, and not enough alkaline foods to counteract them. Some forms of arthritis are created by an allergic reaction to alkaloids found in nightshade vegetables and even nicotine. Not everyone has this allergy, but stopping the consumption of these certain foods could help diagnose the problem.

High Oxalate - Kidney stones

Oxalates are a natural part of most plant foods. It is said that Mother Nature included them in plants as a natural protection from bugs. They are an oxidant that easily forms free radicals in the body. Oxalates are one component of kidney stones. If a person tends to have kidney stones, then reducing the amount of high oxalate foods may help. Other factors include lack of water intake, high calcium, and high consumption of refined foods, which explains why they occur ten times more often than 100 years ago.

Suppresses Thyroid

Someone diagnosed with hypothyroidism (an underactive thyroid) should definitely avoid certain foods. These are natural foods that contain a substance called goitrogens which block the absorption of iodine needed for the thyroid. These should be eaten by those diagnosed with hyperthyroidism.

FOOD HEALTH FACTOR REFERENCE CHART

These are common attributes of certain foods to be aware of.

Top Food Allergies	Acid	Alkaline	Anti-Inflam	Inflam-matory	High Glycemic Not For Diabetics	High Purines - adds to Gout	Inflames Arthritis	High Oxalate - Kidney Stones	Suppress Thyroid
FRUITS									
Acerola Cherries		X	X+						
Apples		X	X	X					X
Apricots		X	X	X					
Avocado		X	X						
Bananas (green)	X		X	X	X				
Bananas (ripe)		X	X		X				
Blackberries		X	X					X	
Blueberries		X	X	X				X	
Boysenberries		X	X	X				X	
Cantaloupe		X	X						
Casaba Melon		X	X	X					
Cherries		X	X**						
Coconut		X	X						
Cranberries	X		X	X					
Dates	X		X	X	X				
Dried Fruits (not raisins)	X		X	X	X	X			
Figs	X		X	X	X			X	
Fruit Juices		X		X	X+		X		
Grapefruit		X	X						X
Grapes		X	X	X	X			X purple	

FOOD HEALTH FACTOR REFERENCE CHART

These are common attributes of certain foods to be aware of.

Food	Acid	Alkaline	Anti-Inflam	Inflam-matory	High Glycemic - Not For Diabetics	High Purines - adds to Gout	Inflames Arthritis	High Oxalate - Kidney Stones	Suppress Thyroid
Guavas	X								
Huckleberries		X	X						
Kiwi		X	X	X				X	
Kumquat		X	X						
Lemons		X	X						
Limes		X	X						
Loganberries		X	X	X					
Mango		X	X	X	X				
Melons		X	X						
Mulberries		X	X						
Nectarine		X	X	X					
Oranges		X	X	X					
Papaya		X	X	X	X				
Passionfruit		X	X	X					
Peaches		X	X	X					X
Pears		X	X	X	X				
Persimmons		X	X						
Pineapple		X	X	X					
Plantains	X			X					
Plums	X		X	X					
Pomegranates	X								

FOOD HEALTH FACTOR REFERENCE CHART

These are common attributes of certain foods to be aware of.

Food	Acid	Alkaline	Anti-Inflam	Inflam-matory	High Glycemic Not For Diabetics	High Purines - adds to Gout	Inflames Arthritis	High Oxalate - Kidney Stones	Suppress Thyroid
Prunes	X				X				
Raisins		X		X	X				
Raspberries, Red		X	X						
Raspberries, Black		X	X					X	
Rhubarb	X		X					X	
Strawberries		X	X					X	X
Tangerines		X	X	X				X	
Tomato									
Watermelon		X	X	X	X				

FOOD HEALTH FACTOR REFERENCE CHART

These are common attributes of certain foods to be aware of.

Food	Acid	Alkaline	Anti-Inflam	Inflammatory	High Sugar/ Glycemic Load	High Purines - Inflames Gout	Inflames Arthritis	High Oxalate - Kidney Stones	Suppress Thyroid	Foods That May Cause Allergies
VEGETABLES										
Alfalfa Sprouts		X	X							
Artichoke		X	X							
Arugula		X	X							
Asparagus		X	X			X				
Avocado		X	X+							
Bamboo Shoots		X	X							
Bean Sprouts		X	X							
Beets		X	X					X++		
Bell Peppers		X	X							
Bok Choy		X	X							
Broccoli		X	X						X	
Brussel Sprouts		X	X					X	X	
Cabbage		X	X						X	
Carrots		X	X+							
Cauliflower		X	X			X			X	
Celery		X	X					X		
Chili Peppers		X	X+							X
Coconut		X	X	X						
Collard Greens		X	X+					X	X	
Corn	X			X					X	X

FOOD HEALTH FACTOR REFERENCE CHART

These are common attributes of certain foods to be aware of.

Food	Acid	Alkaline	Anti-Inflam	Inflam-matory	High Sugar/ Glycemic Load	High Purines - Inflames Gout	Inflames Arthritis	High Oxalate - Kidney Stones	Suppress Thyroid	Foods That May Cause Allergies
Cucumber		X	X							
Dandelion Greens		X	X							
Eggplant		X	X				X			
Endive/Escarole		X	X							
Garlic		X	X							X
Green Beans		X	X					X		
Green Pepper		X	X				X	X		
Grits, white corn	X			X				X		X
Kale		X	X+					X	X	
Leeks		X	X+					X		
Lettuce		X	X							
Lima Beans	X			X					X	
Mushrooms		X	X			X				
Mustard Greens		X	X					X	X	
Okra		X	X					X		
Onions		X	X+						X	
Parsley		X	X					X		
Parsnips		X		X						
Peas		X	X			X				
Pepper, Jalapeno		X	X							X
Pepper, Red		X	X							

FOOD HEALTH FACTOR REFERENCE CHART

These are common attributes of certain foods to be aware of.

Food	Acid	Alkaline	Anti-Inflam	Inflam-matory	High Glycemic Not For Diabetics	High Purines - adds to Gout	May Inflame Arthritis	High Oxalate - Kidney Stones	Suppress Thyroid	Foods That May Cause Allergies
Pepper, Serrano		X	X+							X
Pepper, Yellow		X	X+							
Popcorn	X			X			X			
Potatoes, no skin	X			X			X	X		
Potatoes, with skin		X		X			X	X		
Potatoes Sweet		X	X				X	X		
Pumpkin		X	X					X		
Radicchio		X	X					X		
Radish		X	X							
Rhubarb		X	X					X++		
Rutabaga		X	X					X	X	
Sauerkraut		X	X						X	
Seaweed		X	X							
Spaghetti Squash		X	X							
Spinach		X	X			X		X		X
Summer Squash		X	X					X		
Sweet Potato / Yams		X	X					X	X	
Swiss Chard		X	X					X		
Tomatoes	X	X								X
Tomatoes, Stewed				X			X			X
Turnips		X	X						X	

FOOD HEALTH FACTOR REFERENCE CHART

These are common attributes of certain foods to be aware of.

Food	Acid	Alkaline	Anti-Inflam	Inflam-matory	High Glycemic Not For Diabetics	High Purines - adds to Gout	May Inflame Arthritis	High Oxalate - Kidney Stones	Suppress Thyroid	Foods That May Cause Allergies
Turnip Greens		X	X					X		
Water Chestnuts		X	X							
Watercress		X	X					X	X	
Zucchini		X	X							

FOOD HEALTH FACTOR REFERENCE CHART

These are common attributes of certain foods to be aware of.

Food	Acid	Alkaline	Anti-Inflam	Inflam-matory	High Sugar/Glycemic Load	High Purines - Inflames Gout	Inflames Arthritis	High Oxalate - Kidney Stones	Suppress Thyroid	Foods That May Cause Allergies
Meats/Fish										
Beef, Grain-Fed	X			X		X	X			
Beef, Grass-Fed	X		X			X				
Ground Meat	X			X		X	X			
Chicken	X			X		X				
Cornish Hens	X			X		X				
Duck	X		X			X				
Game	X			X		X				
Goose	X		X			X				
Lamb	X			X		X				
Organ Meat	X			X		X	X			
Turkey	X			X		X	X			
Pork	X		X			X	X			
Veal	X			X		X	X			
Shellfish	X		X			X			X	X
Farmed Fish/Salmon	X			X		X	X			X
Wild Salmon	X		X			X				X
Sushi w/white rice	X		X							X
Swordfish	X					X			X	
Tuna	X					X			X	X
Freshwater Fish	X					X			X	

FOOD HEALTH FACTOR REFERENCE CHART

These are common attributes of certain foods to be aware of.

Food	Acid	Alkaline	Anti-Inflam	Inflam-matory	High Sugar/Glycemic Load	Inflames Gout	Inflames Arthritis	High Oxalate	Suppress Thyroid	Foods That May Cause Allergies
Grain Foods/Flour										
Alfalfa, sprouted			X				X			
Amaranth	X			X				X		
100% Whole Wheat Fl.	X			X			X	X	X	X
Barley	X			X			X			X
Breads/Pastries	X			X						X
Buckwheat	X			X						
Bulgur	X			X			X			
Cereals	X			X						X
Corn/Maize/Tortillas	X			X					X	X
Cornmeal	X			X+					X	X
Couscous	X			X						
Durum	X			X+			X		X	X
Flour Tortillas, white	X			X					X	X
Flr Tortillas, whole grn	X			X					X	X
Graham Crackers/Flour	X			X				X	X	X
Grits/Hominy	X			X				X	X	X
Kamut	X			X			X			
Oat Bran	X			X						X
Oat/Oatmeal		X		X						X

FOOD HEALTH FACTOR REFERENCE CHART

These are common attributes of certain foods to be aware of.

Food	Acid	Alkaline	Anti-Inflam	Inflam-matory	High Sugar/Glycemic Load	Inflames Gout	Inflames Arthritis	High Oxalate-Kidney Stones	Suppress Thyroid	Foods That May Cause Allergies
Pasta, refined	X			X						X
Pasta, whole grain	X									X
Popcorn								X		X
Potato Flour	X			X						
Quinoa		X		X						
Rice/Flour, Brown	X			X						
Rice/Flour, White	X			X						
Rye	X			X			X			X
Semolina (durum flour)	X			X			X			X
Spelt							X	X		
Sprouted Grains	X			X						X
Soy	X			X				X		X
Tapioca Flour	X			X						
Triticale				X			X			
Wheat Bran, Germ	X			X				X		
White Flour	X			X						
White Rice	X			X						X
Whole Wheat Pasta	X			X				X		X
Whole Wheat Tortillas	X			X				X		X
Wild Rice		X		X						

FOOD HEALTH FACTOR REFERENCE CHART

These are common attributes of certain foods to be aware of.

Food	Acid	Alkaline	Anti-Inflam	Inflam-matory	High Sugar/ Glycemic Load	Inflames Gout	Inflames Arthritis	High Oxalate	Suppress Thyroid	Foods That May Cause Allergies
Nuts/Seeds										
Almonds		X	X					X		X
Brazil Nuts			X							X
Cashews		X	X							X
Chestnuts		X		X						
Flaxseed		X	X							
Hazelnuts/Filberts	X		X							
Macadamia Nuts		X	X							X
Peanuts	X		X			X		X	X	X
Pecans	X		X					X		X
Pine Nuts	X			X					X	X
Pistachio Nuts	X		X							X
Poppy Seeds				X						
Pumpkin Seeds		X		X				X		
Sesame Seeds		X		X						X
Soybeans / Nuts/Tofu	X			X				X	X	X
Sunflower Seeds		X		X				X		X
Walnuts	X			X					X	X

FOOD HEALTH FACTOR REFERENCE CHART

These are common attributes of certain foods to be aware of.

Food	Acid	Alkaline	Anti-Inflam	Inflam-matory	High Glycemic Not For Diabetics	High Purines - adds to Gout	May Inflame Arthritis	High Oxalate - Kidney Stones	Suppress Thyroid	Foods That May Cause Allergies
Eggs/Cheese/Dairy										
Eggs		X		X						X
Cheese	X			X			X			X
Cottage Cheese	X		X				X			X
Cream	X			X			X			X
Milk	X			X			X			X
Sour Cream	X			X			X			X
Yogurt - Plain, w/ sugar	X			X			X			X
Grass-Fed Milk Products		X	X							X
Butter	X			X						X
Butter, Ghee	X	X								X
Whey, cow and goat		X		X			X			X

FOOD HEALTH FACTOR REFERENCE CHART

These are common attributes of certain foods to be aware of.

Food	Acid	Alkaline	Anti-Inflam	Inflam-matory	High Sugar/ Glycemic Load	Inflames Gout	Inflames Arthritis	High Oxalate	Suppress Thyroid	Foods That May Cause Allergies
Beans/Legumes										
Baked Beans	X			X		X		X		
Black/Red Beans	X			X		X				
Black Eyed Peas	X			X		X				
Bean Sprouts		X	X							
Butter Beans	X			X		X				
Chickpea/Garbanzo	X			X		X		X		
Edamame	X			X		X				
Fava Beans	X			X		X				
Green Beans/Snap		X	X	X		X				
Kidney Beans	X			X		X				
Lentils		X	X			X				
Lima Beans	X			X		X				
Mung Beans	X			X		X				
Navy Beans	X			X		X				
Peanuts/Peanut Butter	X			X		X				X
Pinto Beans	X			X		X				
Snap Peas						X		X		
Soybeans	X			X		X		X	X	X
Split Peas	X			X		X				

FOOD HEALTH FACTOR REFERENCE CHART

These are common attributes of certain foods to be aware of.

Food	Acid	Alkaline	Anti-Inflam	Inflam-matory	High Sugar/Glycemic Load	Inflames Gout	Inflames Arthritis	High Oxalate	Suppress Thyroid	Foods That May Cause Allergies
Oils/Fats										
Almond Oil	X		X							
Avocado Oil		X	X							
Butter	X			X						
Canola Oil	X		X						X	
Cocoa Butter	X			X						
Coconut Oil		X		X						
Cod Liver Oil		X	X++							
Corn Oil	X			X					X	
Cottonseed Oil	X			X						
Fish Oil	X		X++						X	
Flax Oil		X	X							
Grape Seed Oil	X			X						
Hazelnut Oil	X		X							
Lard	X			X		X				
Margarine		X		X						
Olive Oil		X	X							
Palm/Palm Kernel Oil		X		X						
Peanut Oil	X			X						X

FOOD HEALTH FACTOR REFERENCE CHART

These are common attributes of certain foods to be aware of.

Food	Acid	Alkaline	Anti-Inflam	Inflam-matory	High Sugar/ Glycemic Load	Inflames Gout	Inflames Arthritis	High Oxalate	Suppress Thyroid	Foods That May Cause Allergies
Safflower Oil	X			X						
Safflower -High Oleic	X		X						X	
Sesame Oil	X			X						X
Shortening	X			X						
Soybean Oil	X			X					X	
Sunflower Oil	X			X					X	X
Walnut Oil	X			X					X	
Wheat Germ Oil	X			X						X

FOOD HEALTH FACTOR REFERENCE CHART

These are common attributes of certain foods to be aware of.

Food	Acid	Alkaline	Anti-Inflam	Inflam-matory	High Glycemic Not For Diabetics	High Purines - adds to Gout	May Inflame Arthritis	High Oxalate - Kidney Stones	Suppress Thyroid	Foods That May Cause Allergies
Beverages										
Beer	X			X		X	X	X		X
Coffee (Plain)	X		X				X		X	
Fruit Juices		X		X	X	X	X			
Fruit Juice, Berry		X		X	X	X	X	X		
Gatorade	X			X	X	X	X			
Milk	X			X			X		X	X
Ovaltine	X			X	X	X	X	X	X	
Sodas	X			X	X	X	X			
Soy Milk	X			X					X	X
Tea	X		X					X		
Wine	X		X						X	X
Club Soda		X	X							
Alcohol	X		X	X					X	
Coconut Milk/Water		X	X			X				
Almond Milk		X	X							X
Rice Milk	X									
Mineral Water		X								

FOOD HEALTH FACTOR REFERENCE CHART

These are common attributes of certain foods to be aware of.

Food	Acid	Alkaline	Anti-Inflam	Inflam-matory	High Glycemic Not For Diabetics	High Purines - adds to Gout	May Inflame Arthritis	High Oxalate - Kidney Stones	Suppress Thyroid	Foods That May Cause Allergies
Condiments/Sauce										
Apple Cider Vinegar		X	X							
Hot Sauce	X		X							X
Jam/Jelly	X			X						
Mayonnaise	X			X						
Mustard	X		X							
Salad Dressings	X			X						
Salsa, w/white vinegar	X			X						
Salsa, w/ac vinegar	X		X							
Soy Sauce, w/wheat	X		X	X				X		X
Soy Sauce, w/o wheat	X							X		X
Vinegar, white	X			X						
Worcestershire	X			X						

FOOD HEALTH FACTOR REFERENCE CHART

These are common attributes of certain foods to be aware of.

Food Herbs/Spices	Acid	Alkaline	Anti-Inflam	Inflam-matory	High Sugar/Glycemic Load	Inflames Gout	Inflames Arthritis	High Oxalate	Suppress Thyroid	Foods That May Cause Allergies
Allspice		X	X							
Basil		X	X							
Bay Leaf		X	X							
Black Pepper		X	X					X		
Capers			X							
Caraway Seeds		X	X							
Cardamom		X	X							
Cayenne		X	X++							
Celery Seeds		X	X							
Chervil		X	X							
Chili Pepper/Powder		X	X++							X
Chives		X	X							
Cilantro		X	X							
Cinnamon		X	X					X		
Cloves		X	X							
Coriander		X	X							
Cumin		X	X							
Curry Powder	X		X++							
Dill		X	X							
Fennel		X	X							

FOOD HEALTH FACTOR REFERENCE CHART

These are common attributes of certain foods to be aware of.

Food	Acid	Alkaline	Anti-Inflam	Inflam-matory	High Sugar/Glycemic Load	Inflames Gout	Inflames Arthritis	High Oxalate	Suppress Thyroid	Foods That May Cause Allergies
Garlic/Garlic Powder		X	X++							X
Ginger		X	X++					X		
Lemongrass		X	X							
Lemon Peel		X	X							
Mace		X	X							
Marjoram		X	X							
Mint		X	X							
Mustard Seed		X	X							
Nutmeg		X		X						
Onion Powder		X	X++							
Oregano		X	X							
Paprika		X	X							
Parsley		X	X							
Rosemary		X	X							
Saffron		X	X							
Sage		X	X							
Salt	X									
Sea Salt		X	X							
Tarragon		X	X							
Thyme		X	X							
Turmeric		X	X++							

FOOD HEALTH FACTOR REFERENCE CHART

These are common attributes of certain foods to be aware of.

Food	Acid	Alkaline	Anti-Inflam	Inflam-matory	High Glycemic Not For Diabetics	High Purines - adds to Gout	May Inflame Arthritis	High Oxalate - Kidney Stones	Suppress Thyroid	Foods That May Cause Allergies
Sweeteners										
Agave	X			X		X	X		X	
Brown Sugar	X			X	X	X	X		X	
Brown Rice Syrup		X		X	X					
Corn Syrup	X			X	X	X	X			
Equal//Sweet n Low	X			X		X	X			
Fructose	X			X	X	X	X			
Hich Fructose Corn Syr.	X++			X++	X	X	X		X	X
Honey, commercial	X			X	X	X	X			
Honey, Raw		X	X							
Maple Syrup	X			X		X	X			
Malt	X			X	X	X	X			
Maltodextrin	X			X	X	X	X			
Splenda	X			X		X	X			
Stevia		X	X							
Sucanat		X	X							
Sucralose	X			X		X	X			
White/Refined Sugar	X			X	X	X	X		X	
Xylitol		X	X							
Chocolate (commercial)	X			X			X	X		
Raw Chocolate		X		X			X	X		

Chapter 10

Transition Recipes

These recipes are common, yet incorporate new ways of cooking in order to avoid refined foods and high-heat cooking. Food is how we survive, and is a precious commodity that needs to be treated with respect: no high heat or frying, no refinement, etc. Ultimately eating more raw foods is highly important. The foods we choose to eat pass through the center of our immune system, and provide the nutrition each food ultimately possesses; our choices in eating and cooking are critical.

-The way we treat our food is just as critical as the way we treat our body-

Before Following Recipes...

Never cook on the stove at temps higher than the medium setting.
Most foods cook fine on very low heat.

When using **dried spices**, add a small amount of water to them in a bowl to rehydrate and help bring out the flavor.

Thickening Options:
Arrowroot makes a nice thickener for sauces, but it cannot be boiled once it is incorporated. It thickens on its own in the hot mixture.

Potato or whole grain flours make good thickening agents instead of typical white flour or cornstarch.

Sugars

When *sugar* is listed in recipes, there are several options available for replacing refined white sugar. Experiment with these more natural, more harmonious sugars, and find a preference. Choose from these following natural substitutes:

- Coconut Sugar (a brown sugar)
- Coconut Nectar (like honey)
- Sucanat (natural brown sugar)
- Xylitol (white sugar; birch source is the best)
- Erythritol (white sugar, not as sweet; requires 1:2 ratio)
- Luo Han (1:25 ratio) (similar to stevia)
- Stevia (1:20 ratio)
- Raw honey (uncooked recipes only)
- Maple Syrup
- Ripe Banana
- Homemade Applesauce w/skin/jarred unsweetened applesauce

Combination of sugars can be used. I recommend alternating and combining sugar sources whenever possible.

When using banana or applesauce, oil content can also be cut in half, since the fruit is full of natural moisture.

Xylitol is very nutritious, good for diabetics, kills bad bacteria, and treats gum disease, but be aware that xylitol and erythritol can cause diarrhea if used in excess;1 TBLS per serving 1-2 times a day is within limits for most people. Most times half xylitol and half stevia or another sugar can be used in a recipe.

*Also, because a dog's pancreas (unlike a human's) releases a potent amount of insulin when xylitol is ingested, it can be fatal to dogs.

Oils

Only use expeller-pressed, extra virgin, or cold-pressed versions of these oils:
- Olive
- Coconut
- Sunflower
- Flax *(only use for uncooked recipes)*

Combinations of oils can be used.
Try to substitute at least 1/4 of oil in recipes with coconut oil, since coconut oil has extremely high nutritional qualities, yet has a strong flavor.

Keep in mind that all cooking oils are again another processed food. Since the oils are extracted from the main food product, usually nuts and seeds, they are not a whole food. Try to limit the use of all cooking oils; suggestions for substitution include: natural applesauce (containing peel), whole avocado, almond/nut butters, or just water.

Flax oil should only be used for non-cooked recipes, such as salad dressings because of its high omega 3 content, which is so important that it should not be destroyed by heating.

Any oils can easily become oxidized when heated to very high temperatures, forming free radicals, especially when used over and over.

Basically, there is not getting around avoiding free radicals. Check the charts at the end of the book to find the foods with high natural antioxidants to counteract these free radicals.

Combination of oils can be used in some recipes.

Dairy

I strongly recommend dairy be avoided. Through years of study, I continue to find reasons that it just is not conducive with the human body. Dairy proteins have been found to possibly be the cause of various allergies, and a contributor to many autoimmune disorders; the effect can be so subtle or hidden that this as the cause can go undetected, yet trigger major disorder or disease oriented side effects. Studies indicate it may be the root cause of Type 1 diabetes, multiple sclerosis, asthma, breast cancer, menopausal hot flashes, and many more disorders. But more common effects are asthma, allergies, and lactose intolerance.

If the use of dairy is desired, the only dairy products to consider in recipes in limited amounts for flavor purposes (and if you have no health issues), would be:

Raw Parmigiano-Reggiano
Raw goat milk/cheese
Raw grass-fed butter
Nothing else.

However, these should never be cooked because they would lose their enzymes.

Alternative Milks

There are several types of milk substitutes to replace cow's milk in recipes. Made from nuts and grains, they are lactose free. Some work better with hot foods, some work better with cold.

Always choose the UNSWEETENED form of any alternative milk. Almond and Cashew milk can be easily made at home (recipes are in this chapter). Most commercial milks contain an additive called carrageenan, which is under scrutiny as having allergic reactions, side effects. Some milks, such as brown rice milk, have brands without the additive. Making almond or cashew milk at home will guarantee an additive-free product.

Almond	– *alkaline, breaks down in cooked recipes*
Brown Rice	– *high natural sugar*
Cashew *(thickest)*	– *taste most similar to cow's milk*
	works the best for cream replacement;
	taste is creamy; sauces will be thicker
Coconut *(thicker)*	– *does not have a distinct coconut flavor*
	works well in hot or cold recipes
Flax	– *nice flavor, good Omega 3, not for cooked dishes*
Hemp Milk	– *odd taste, good protein*
Oat	– *high protein, alkaline*
Soy Milk	– *highly allergic*
Sunflower	– *nice flavor, high Vit. E, w/sunflower lecithin*

Baking with Flour

For the recipes calling for flour, 100% whole-wheat flour can be used, or any combinations of these flours. Whole wheat is a heavy substance, so combining with a lighter flour (gluten-free) such as oat, will create a lighter product.

Gluten-free flours are:

Almond	Quinoa
Buckwheat	Amaranth
Coconut	Tapioca
Oat	Sorghum
Brown rice	

Gluten Flours are:

Wheat	Rye
Barley	Spelt
Kamut	Durum
Bulgur	Semolina
Triticale	

Using less gluten flours, especially wheat, will contribute to better health, as the gluten in wheat has been intensified by GMO procedures and modern growing techniques.

**When using all gluten-free flour, add 1/2 tsp of xanthan gum powder for each cup of flour. (*corn-free xanthan gum is available.*)

Add a TBLS of a natural fiber additive like *Garden of Life SuperSeed* whenever possible for added fiber and nutrients.

COOKED GRAINS/SEEDS

These simple foods are easily cooked as follows, and great for adding all kinds of fruits and vegetables for some delicious wholesome dishes:
*Always keep lid on pan until completely cooked.

Quinoa (keen-wa)
(great side dish; alkaline food; actually a seed)

1 cup quinoa
2-1/4 cups water

Bring water to a boil
Add quinoa and cover
Reduce heat to low
Cook for 20 minutes, and remove from heat
Let sit for 10 minutes before serving or using

Brown (Red, Black, Wild) Rice
(great side dish; acidic)

1 cup brown rice
2-1/4 cups water

Bring water to a boil
Add rice and cover
Reduce heat to low
Cook for 40 minutes, and remove from heat
Let sit for 10 minutes before serving or using

Amaranth

(great hot cereal; alkaline food)

1 cup amaranth
3 cups water
 (some prefer 2/3 cup per each 2 cups water; your preference)

Bring water to a boil
Add amaranth and cover; Reduce heat to low
Cook for 25 minutes, and remove from heat
Let sit covered for 10 minutes before serving or using

Oatmeal

(great hot cereal; alkaline food)

1 cup oatmeal
2-1/2 - 3 cups water

Bring water to a boil
Add oatmeal
Reduce heat to low
Cook for 20 minutes, cover, and remove from heat
Let sit for 10 minutes before serving or using

MAKE YOUR OWN CONDIMENTS

Mayonnaise *(basis for many dressings)*

1 Egg
1/4 tsp mustard powder
1-1/2 tsp wine vinegar or apple cider vinegar
2 TBLS lemon juice
1/8 tsp Salt – Pepper

Mix all ingredients above

DO NOT ADD OIL ALL AT ONCE – follow this direction:
1 Cup expeller-pressed olive and/or sunflower oil
Add 1 cup oil *EXTREMELY* slow while mixture is blending.

Ketchup

1 cup plain Tomato Sauce (1 small 8 oz. can)
1 TBLS Apple Cider Vinegar
1 TBLS Sucanat
1/2 tsp sea salt
1 tsp xylitol
1/2 tsp. Arrowroot

Mix all ingredients together in saucepan
Heat on low heat for two minutes; do not let it boil

Mustard

1/4 cup Mustard Powder
2 TBLS Raw Apple Cider Vinegar
1/3 cup Water
1/4 Tsp Turmeric

Heat only to warm to dissolve mustard powder
Stir and let sit for 1 hour to dissolve mustard powder
Mixture will thicken with time
Stir, refrigerate (thin with water as you see fit)

Make Your Own Cashew Milk (or almond)

1 cup raw cashews
Soak in a bowl of water for 4-6 hours
Drain and rinse

Place cashews and 3 cups water into a blender
Blend for 1-3 minutes

Cashew milk is a newcomer to milk alternatives,
and very, very tasty. It has such a rich, creamy texture that it
can be a great substitute for cream

You now have your own cashew milk; a great substitute for
cow milk, and a little creamier than coconut and almond milk
Be sure to use a wide-mouth container for storing cashew
milk; it adheres somewhat to the sides of the container,
making it difficult to clean.
(keeps for 10 days)

Make Your Own Margarine

1/2 cup coconut milk *(unsweetened, in the carton, not canned)*
1 tsp raw apple cider vinegar
1/2 tsp sea salt
2 tsp raw *sunflower lecithin
1/2 tsp xanthan gum
1/4 tsp turmeric
2/3 cup raw organic coconut oil
1/3 cup flaxseed oil
1/3 cup virgin olive oil or sunflower oil

Combine milk and apple cider vinegar to ferment
(Let sit 15 min.)
Add salt, lecithin, xanthan gum, turmeric to milk, and mix
Put into blender
Combine oils in a pouring container
Turn on the blender to slow, and add the oil slowly; when all
oil is in, turn up the blender to high to whip
Pour into glass containers

**Sunflower lecithin can be found online; eg.,
mysunflowerlecitin.com*

It can also be taken daily as a nutritional supplement.

SALADS

For recipes asking for mayonnaise, only use homemade mayonnaise, or these current brands: Earth Balance (soy-free) or Trader Joe's Yellow Label (or the like). **Never use any other commercial mayonnaise** *(unless it meets the criteria for healthful), and never use more than 1 TBLS mayonnaise per serving/per person*

GREEN Tuna (or Wild Salmon) Salad

1 Can Tuna (or wild salmon), drained
2 tsp lemon juice - sprinkle on tuna
1 stalk celery – diced
2 cups thinly sliced or chopped cabbage
2 chopped green onions
1/4 cup chopped parsley or cilantro (optional)
Chopped walnuts (optional pumpkin seeds or almonds)
4-6 green olives (w/or without pimento), chopped
1 chopped dill pickle (optional)
2 – 3 TBLS Mayonnaise
salt – pepper

Combine all ingredients; chill
Makes 2-3 servings
Requires no bread

Mediterranean Salad

1 chopped cucumber
½ cup Chopped onion
1 cup Chopped red cabbage (or green)
1 Diced Tomato
2 TBLS chopped Parsley
1 TBLS chopped Cilantro
1 diced celery
1/3 cup Garbanzo beans
1 clove chopped Garlic
1 TBLS olive oil
1 TBLS apple cider vinegar
1 TBLS lemon juice
1/ 4 tsp Black pepper
Use any or all ingredients

Warm Spinach Salad

Spinach, 1 whole package or bunch
1 cup Bean sprouts
2 TBLS Extra virgin olive oil
2 TBLS red wine vinegar (or apple cider vinegar or balsamic)
1-2 clove garlic chopped
2 tsp. Raw Honey
1/2 cup thinly sliced sweet onions

Combine vinegar, garlic and olive oil in pan; heat
Add spinach and bean sprouts, heat together for just 1 minute
Remove from heat and mix in honey
Place on plate and top with slivered raw onion

Avocado Salad

2-3 ripe avocadoes, diced
1/2 cup chopped red onion
1/2 cup chopped tomato
1/2 cup cubed cucumber
1/2 cup mashed berries
(raspberries/strawberries/blackberries)
　　　mix with 1 TBLS fresh lemon juice
Fresh basil or cilantro, chopped
1/3 cup walnuts, almonds or pine nuts

Mix all together, chill, serve

Simple Cole Slaw

3-4 cups shredded, sliced or chopped cabbage
　　　　　(optional 1/4 cup grated carrot)
2 TBLS homemade or recommended mayonnaise
1-2 TBLS apple cider vinegar or fresh lemon juice
1/8 tsp black pepper

Mix vinegar and mayonnaise together; then add to cabbage
Add pepper, mix well; chill

Simple Shrimp Salad

4 Large Leaves Green Leaf Lettuce or Romaine, chopped
1/2 large carrot or 1 small, grated
1 cup/can baby shrimp (large shrimp if preferred)
1/2 onion, grated (grate directly into greens for onion juice)
1/4 cup recommended mayonnaise or homemade
1/2 tsp Black Pepper

Mix all together and chill

Seafood Salad

1 cup/can crab meat
1 cup small shrimp
1 stalk celery, sliced
1/4 cup chopped fresh parsley
2 cups shredded green cabbage
1/2 cup shredded red cabbage
1/4 cup homemade or recommended mayonnaise
1 TBLS fresh lemon juice
1/4 tsp Paprika
salt – pepper
1/4 cup chopped mango
1 cup cooked 100% whole-grain elbow macaroni

Cut crab meat into small pieces; mix with shrimp.
Sprinkle lemon juice onto seafood. Mix all ingredients, chill.

SALAD DRESSINGS & SAUCES

True French Dressing

1 egg
1 TBLS paprika
1 TBLS xylitol (optional)
1 tsp salt
1/8 tsp cayenne
1 TBL raw honey
1/2 tsp garlic powder
1/2 cup apple cider and/or wine vinegar

Add all but the oil; beat well. Add oil slowly while blending
-- 1 cup olive oil and/or any other expeller-pressed oil
Mix in blender for 20-30 seconds

Simple Everyday Oil & Vinegar Dressing

1 cup Olive and/or Flaxseed Oil
1/2 cup Fresh Lemon Juice and/or Apple Cider Vinegar
1/2 cup Balsamic Vinegar
2 TBLS water
1 TBLS Paprika
1 tsp mustard powder
1/2 tsp garlic powder

Mix all ingredients together by shaking in bottle or blending
For creamy oil and vinegar, add 2 TBLS mayonnaise

Ranch Dressing

2 tsp. apple cider vinegar
2 tsp. lemon juice
1 cup Recommended mayonnaise or homemade

Add vinegar and lemon juice to mayo and let sit
15 minutes to ferment.
Add any or all remaining ingredients below, to your taste:

1 tsp. garlic powder
1/2 tsp. salt
1/4 tsp. fresh pepper
1 tsp. fresh or dried parsley
1 TBLS Parmesan (optional)
1 tsp. water
1/2 tsp dried chives
1/2 tsp dried dill weed
1/4 tsp onion powder

Quick French Dressing

1 cup recommended mayonnaise or homemade
1 TBLS Paprika
1/2 tsp garlic powder
1 TBLS apple cider vinegar
1 TBLS lemon juice
2 TBLS water
1/8 tsp dry mustard powder (optional)
For Thousand Island: add 1 TBLS pickle relish or chopped pickles

Fish Marinade

2 TBLS olive oil
Juice of one lemon
1/4 cup Tamari soy sauce
2 TBLS balsamic vinegar
1/4 cup Marsala wine
1/2 tsp mustard powder
1 tsp garlic powder
1 tsp brown rice syrup

Mix all together
Mix 1 tsp arrowroot w/1/4 cup coconut milk
Add to marinade for thickening

Hollandaise Sauce

3 egg yolks
2 TBLS water
1 TBLS lemon juice
1/3 cup oil blend (olive/coconut, or raw butter)
1/2 tsp salt
Pinch of Cayenne (to taste)

Put all ingredients together into a saucepan except
oil/butter
Whisk together to thicken, before heating
Turn on heat to low, whisking continually, to a
good consistency; do not simmer, only heat

DRINKS

All drinks are prepared in a blender, not a juicer
Only sweeten green or fruit drinks with whole fruits

Energizing Green Drink

1 large leaf romaine, green leaf lettuce, chard or kale
        (or 2 cups spinach)
1/2 cup chopped cucumber
1 carrot
1/3 cup cubed fresh pineapple
1/4 fresh lemon, w/o rind
1/4 cup cubed watermelon rind (optional...good for detox)
1/3 cup water or coconut water
Blend till smooth; add 1 cup+ ice; blend till smooth

Cleansing Fruit Smoothie

1/2 banana
1/2 cup diced pineapple
1 cup kale or spinach
1/4 cup parsley
1/4 cup coconut water
Blend on high for 1 - 2 minutes
Add 1 cup ice
Blend for 30 seconds

Berry Smoothie

1/2 cup raspberries
1/2 cup blueberries
1 TBLS fresh lemon
1/2 cup chopped kale or spinach leaves
1/2 cup water
1/4 cup alternative milk or 1/3 banana (optional)
1/2 cup ice

Healthy Orange Julius Smoothie
Makes a meal **(1 Serving)**

1 Large Orange (or 2 small), meat of complete inside
2 tsp xylitol
1 tsp real vanilla extract
1/4 cup alternative milk
Mix until smooth

Add:
1 raw egg
1/4 cup alternative milk
Mix only a few seconds

Add:
1 cup ice; MIX till ice is dissolved (20 seconds)

Cold Chocolate Drink

1 cup alternative milk - unsweetened
1 tsp Xylitol
1 tsp Coconut sugar
1-3 tsp natural raw cacao/cocoa powder
1 tsp. natural vanilla extract (optional)
Blend
Pour over ice
FOR BLENDED FROSTY smoothie:
Add and blend ½-1 cup ice cubes

Iced Mocha

Heat 1/4 cup water to steep 1-3 tsp organic coffee grounds
Pour water over grounds in coffee filter
Add 1 tsp cacao to warm coffee
1 tsp Xylitol
1 tsp Coconut sugar
1/2 cup coconut milk
Blend, cool
Pour over ice

Hot Chocolate

Mix cocoa and xylitol together in cooking pan
Add small amount of milk to dissolve cacao
Turn on low heat
Add rest of milk; mix and heat to low simmer; do not boil

Chocolate Malt

1 cup alternative milk
1 TBLS cocoa
1 TBLS xylitol or coconut sugar
1-2 TBLS *malted barley extract powder
1/4 tsp xanthan gum (optional)
2 tsp vanilla

Blend at low speed, then at high for 20 seconds
Add 1 cup ice
Blend for 20 seconds

*Malted barley extract powder can be found online,
such as Aunt Patty's.

Fish Africanz

2 Fish fillets
1 Tomato
2 TBLS red wine or red wine vinegar
1 tsp Curry
1 tsp Turmeric
1/2 tsp Chili powder
1/4 tsp Cumin
1/4 tsp garlic powder
1 garlic clove, chopped
1/4 cup coconut milk
1 thinly sliced (red) onion

Place fish in shallow, oiled sauté pan
Mix spices and garlic together in 1 TBLS water
Spread onto fish
Pour coconut milk and wine over fish
Cover fish with sliced tomato and onion
Cover pan, and let simmer on low for 10-15 min.
Or bake 30 min. @ 350 degrees

Cabbage Rolls

12 large cabbage leaves
1 cup cooked brown rice or quinoa
1 egg
1-1/4 lb. Ground chicken/turkey
2 tsp Salt
1/2 tsp pepper
1/2 onion chopped
1 tsp Poultry seasoning
Sauce:

> 3 cups tomato sauce
> 1 Tbls. Sucanat
> 1 Tbls. Lemon juice
> 1/4 cup water

Soak leaves in boiled water until limp (or in steamer)
Fill cabbage leaves and roll
Secure with toothpicks
Place half of sauce on bottom of pan
Place cabbage rolls in pan and cover
Cook for 1 hour on low heat

Nut Crusted Baked Salmon

4 Wild Salmon Fillets
1 cup crushed almonds
1 cup crushed walnuts
1/8 tsp cayenne pepper
1/2 tsp garlic powder
1/2 tsp ginger
1/2 tsp salt/pepper

1/2 cup coconut milk
2 TBLS olive oil
2 TBLS lemon juice
2 TBLS soy sauce
2 TBLS Marsala wine
1 tsp mustard

Place salmon fillets onto foiled baking pan
Mix dry ingredients; add wet ingredients and mix well
Spread onto top of salmon fillets
Broil for 8 minutes, until salmon is cooked through

Chicken Paprikash

2 TBLS Expeller-pressed oil (to coat pan)
2 Chicken breasts (w/bone or cut up meat), or 4 bone-in
chicken thighs
2 TBLS Paprika
1/2 large onion thinly sliced
1/2 cup sliced red pepper
1 Zucchini, sliced
2-4 tomatoes, chopped
1 cup dry white wine
1 tsp marjoram
salt and pepper to taste
1/2 cup coconut or cashew milk w/1TBLS arrowroot

Coat pan with olive oil
Coat chicken with paprika, salt and pepper, and place pan
Cover with wine; add all other ingredients except milk
Simmer for 30-60 minutes
Remove from heat

Add 1/2 cup coconut or cashew milk mixed with 1 TBLS
arrowroot for thickening

Do not cook further

Chicken Tarragon

Meat of 2 chicken breasts, cut into chunks
2 TBLS olive oil
1 cup chicken broth
1/2 cup Marsala wine
1 cup mushrooms, halved
1/2 onion cut up
1 TBLS brandy (optional)
1 cup coconut milk
2 TBLS tarragon
1 TBLS arrowroot
Garlic

Coat pan with olive oil
Place in pan:
Chicken, broth, Marsala wine, brandy, mushrooms, onion
Cover and cook for 20-30 minutes

Mix together 1 TBLS arrowroot with 2 TBLS coconut milk

Remove chicken from heat
Quickly add garlic, coconut milk, tarragon and arrowroot
Mix to thicken

Turkey Piccata

4 Turkey breast cutlets or breasts
1/2 tsp Salt/pepper
1/2 cup almond flour/ oat flour (flour blend preferred)
2 TBLS olive oil
1/2 cup Marsala wine
1/2 cup water
2 lemons sliced thinly
1 TBLS raw butter or homemade margarine
1/4 cup chopped parsley

Pound turkey to tenderize and flatten
Sprinkle with salt and pepper. Dip turkey in flour
Sauté slowly in oil on low. (Best in a non-stick 'green' pan)
        (Do not allow to brown or sizzle)
Add wine, water, parsley and lemon
Cover and simmer on low for 30-40 minutes.
Remove from heat.

Swirl in butter
Mix 1 TBLS arrowroot w/2 TBLS water;
add to sauce to thicken

Pumpkin Pasta

1/2 cup chicken stock
1/4 cup Marsala/sweet wine
1/2 tsp sea salt
1/4 tsp pepper
1/2 onion thinly sliced
1/2 - 1 yellow squash, sliced
4 diced tomatoes

1/2 cup canned/cooked & mashed pumpkin
1/2 cup alternative milk
1/4 tsp cinnamon
1 TBLS fresh Basil (2 tsp dried)

1 TBLS olive oil

Simmer vegetables, oil, chicken stock, wine, salt/pepper
for 30 minutes
Add pumpkin, cinnamon and basil and alternative milk
Mix and simmer again for 5 minutes
Mix in olive oil
Serve over 100% whole grain/brown rice penne/pasta

Fish on a Bed of Rice

2-3 cups cooked rice
Mix with 1/4 cup canned pumpkin and 1 TBLS lemon juice
   (optional)
1 yellow pepper
1 orange pepper (red pepper optional)
1 lb. fresh cod or any whitefish or wild salmon, etc.

Cut peppers into strips, mix with 2 TBLS expeller-pressed oil
Roast in oven until limp

Cut fish into 1-inch strips
Coat pan with 1 TBLS oil, add fish, cover
Cook for 5-10 minutes
Pour juice of one lemon onto fish

Make Fish Sauce
   (in Salad Dressings and Sauces section above)
Add 2 cloves of chopped garlic

Place a mound of cooked rice on plate
Place cooked fish strips on top of rice
Drizzle with fish sauce
Place roasted peppers on top of fish

Makes 3 or 4 servings

Veggie Burgers

1 cup (or 1 can) mashed, cooked black beans
1/3 cup chopped red or sweet onion
1/4 cup chopped green onion
1/4 cup chopped parsley and/or cilantro
1/3 cup chopped red and/or green pepper
1/2 cup cooked quinoa
1/4 cup grated carrot
2 cloves garlic minced
1/2 tsp paprika powder
1/4 tsp chili powder
1/2 tsp oregano
2 TBLS hot water
2 egg whites
1/4 tsp sea salt

Rinse and drain beans
Heat in saucepan and small amount of water to soften
With gloves on, combine, mix all ingredients with your
hands
Form into patties
Place onto foil-covered pan
Broil at 400, middle rack 6-10 minutes on each side

(may be served with Hollandaise sauce)

SOUPS

Chicken Soup

2 Chicken breasts WITH bones
4 cups chicken broth
4 cups water
2 stalks celery, sliced
1/2 – 1 carrot, grated
1/2 cup chopped parsley
1/2 tsp turmeric
salt/pepper
1/3 cup 100% whole-grain pasta or spaghetti noodles
(broken in 1 inch pieces).

Simmer chicken in broth and water for 1 hour
Remove chicken and allow to cool
Remove bones and skin, and cut chicken into bite-sized
pieces
Return to broth. Add all ingredients except noodles
Simmer for 45 min. Add noodles; cook for 30 min. longer

Chicken bones (as well as skin) add great flavor as well as nutrients, especially from the bone marrow: calcium, magnesium, phosphorous, glycine, etc. These are what contribute to recovery when sick, as it's said that chicken soup should be eaten for flu, etc.; this was meant to include the bones when preparing the soup.

Onion Soup

2-3 large onions sliced thin
1/4 cup butter, olive oil
2 TBLS 100% whole-wheat flour/oat flour
1/4 cup white wine
1 carton beef stock
1 carton chicken stock
4 cups water
1/8 tsp pepper
1/4-1/2 tsp thyme

Place onions in warm pan with butter or oil
Cook 10 minutes on low, stirring occasionally
Add flour – mix well
Add wine – mix well. Add broth, water, spices
Simmer covered for 1 hour

Split Pea Soup

1 cup peas
1 TBLS chopped leek or onion
1 cup chicken broth
2 cups water
1/2 carrot shredded
1 stalk celery – sliced
1/4 tsp Marjoram
dash of oregano
salt-pepper
Simmer all ingredients for 1 hour
Blend soup in blender until smooth

Barley Lentil Soup

1/2 cup lentils
1/4 cup barley
1-2 stalks sliced celery
1 fresh tomato, chopped
1 carton chicken stock
Garlic, 2 cloves, chopped
salt/pepper
clove, nutmeg, 1/4 tsp each
1 cup chopped leek, or 1 onion, chopped

Combine all ingredients, simmer for 45 minutes
Remove from heat
Mix 2 TBLS Arrowroot w/1/2 cup alternative milk or water to thicken
Do not return to heat

Squash Soup

3 cups Butternut, Acorn and/or Pumpkin
  (soak w/1 tsp apple cider vinegar (15 min.)
1 cup chicken broth
2 cups water
1/2 - 1 onion, cut in large pieces
1 carrot, sliced or grated
2 celery stalks, sliced
1/8 tsp nutmeg
1/2 tsp ginger
1/4 tsp cinnamon
1/4 tsp salt

1/2 cup fresh corn
1/2 cup chopped red bell pepper
1 cup cashew or coconut milk

Bake squash in 325 oven until soft, about 1 hour
When cooled, puree in blender with 2 cups water

Mix all other ingredients in pot, except, corn, red pepper, milk
Cook for 40-60 min.

Purée soup mixture in blender
Mix squash and soup mixture in saucepan
Add red bell pepper, corn and milk
Simmer on low 20 minutes longer

SIDE DISHES

French Potatoes

4 large RED potatoes
1/4 cup Olive Oil
1/4 cup red wine vinegar
3 Green onions, chopped into small pieces
2 Cloves garlic, minced
1/2 cup chopped fresh parsley
Black Pepper

DO NOT PEEL potatoes – cut the eyes out, slice thinly
Simmer in water for 5 minutes; do not overcook
Drain, rinse, then chill potatoes for at least 1 hour
Mix together all other ingredients, then add to potatoes
Marinate for 1 hour, stirring lightly, occasionally
Add more oil and vinegar if needed

Broiled Sweet Potato Fries

Cut sweet potato (w/peel) into fry-sized pieces
    (remove bad spots)
Mix potatoes and 1 TBLS expeller-pressed oil in bowl
    (can be made w/o oil, to cut down on oil consumption)

Put potatoes onto paper towel and pat off excess oil. Lay
out cut potatoes onto foil-covered pan. (Use center rack)
Broil for 10-15 minutes, before potatoes start to speckle

Spanish Rice or Quinoa

1/2 cup brown rice or quinoa
1-1/8 cup water
1/2 cup chopped onion
1 tomato puréed (or ¼ cup tomato sauce)
1/2 tomato, diced
Salt/pepper

Combine all ingredients
Bring water to a boil; add all ingredients
Quinoa – Cook covered on low heat for 20 min./Brown rice
40 minutes. Remove from heat, let sit covered 10 min.

Cold Curry Vegetables

1 cup Artichoke hearts
2-3 green onions
2-4 stalks raw asparagus (1 inch removed from ends)
1/4 cup frozen peas
1/2 cup Broccoli cut into small pieces
1 cup orange or yellow peppers, chopped
3 cups cooked brown/colored rice or quinoa, chilled
2 tsp. curry powder
1-2 cloves garlic, minced
1/3 cup recommended mayonnaise or homemade

Chop all veggies and add to chilled rice or quinoa
Add mayonnaise, curry powder, garlic, sea salt, pepper
Mix all together. Add Chopped walnuts (optional)
Serve cold

VEGETABLE DISHES

Ratatouille (ra-ta-too-ee)

2 Zucchini, sliced
1 Eggplant, cubed
1 Red Pepper, diced
1 Onion, sliced or chopped
6 fresh Tomatoes (or 1 large can diced tomatoes)
2 Clove Garlic
1-2 tsp Cumin (ground seeds, not powder)
Salt/pepper

Mix all together and simmer on low, covered, for 30-40 min.

Basque Green Beans

4 cups Green Beans
1/4 cup chopped Red Pepper
2 Cloves Garlic minced
1/2 tsp Oregano (rehydrate dried oregano)
2 TBLS Balsamic Vinegar
2 TBLS Olive Oil
Salt/Pepper to taste
1 large Tomato, diced + 1 more garlic clove minced

Place all ingredients in skillet except Tomato
Sauté on low
Stir and cook for 10 minutes
Add tomato + 1 extra garlic, stir in to reheat

Spinach (or Kale) Cakes

4 cups Spinach or Kale
1/2 cup thinly sliced onion
1 grated zucchini

Place in large skillet;
Heat on low for 5 minutes to remove moisture

Mix together:
2 TBLS almond meal
1/4 cup sprouted grain bread crumbs
2-3 cloves garlic minced
1 TBLS lemon juice
1/2 tsp Nutmeg
1/4 tsp Black pepper
1 tsp Sea salt
1/4 tsp Cayenne
4 Egg whites

Combine mix with vegetables
Form patties (makes 6)
Coat skillet with olive oil
Broil or pan sear on low – 10 minutes each side
   (Do not allow to brown or sizzle)

Make Hollandaise sauce with remaining egg yolks
Top each patty with a spoonful of sauce
(See the Salad Dressing and Sauces section Pg 216)

HORS D'OEUVRES

Stuffed Mild Chiles w/Shrimp

8 Wax Chile peppers (light, yellow/green)
1 cup tiny shrimp and/or crab meat
1/4 cup minced onion
2 cloves garlic, chopped
2 TBLS Lemon Juice
1/3 cup almond meal
1/3 cup chopped cilantro
2 TBLS Olive or sunflower oil
2 TBLS Marsala Wine
2 TBLS *Parmigiano* cheese (optional)

Slowly sautée onion in Marsala wine and oil on low heat
5 minutes
(Wear gloves to prepare chiles; inside oils are very hot)
Cut chilis in half, and pull out center vein and seeds
Mix together all ingredients
Stuff chiles with mixture; Place on baking pan
Cover and bake for 30 min. at 325 degrees
Uncover and broil for 5 minutes

Artichoke Casserole Dip

1 frozen bag or can artichoke hearts (in water) drained and sliced
1/3 cup recommended mayonnaise or homemade
1/4 cup diced mild green chiles
1/2 cup alternative sour cream (w/cashew milk)
1/3 cup *Parmigiano* cheese (optional)
2 cloves minced garlic
1/2 cup sliced, halved (cooked) green beans
1/2 cup cooked/frozen or raw spinach
1/2 cup sliced fresh mushrooms

Mix and place in casserole bowl
Bake 350 degrees – 30 min.

Hummus

1 can garbanzo beans, rinsed and drained, or 2 cups cooked
1/4 cup tahini - unroasted (optional)
2 cloves garlic
4 Tbls olive oil
2 Tbls water
3-4 TBLS lemon juice
1/2 tsp paprika
1/4 tsp sea salt
Dash of Cayenne

Mix in blender or food processor until smooth
Sprinkle paprika on top

Cabbage Roll Appetizers

1/2 lb. ground chicken and ground shrimp
1/4 cup sliced water chestnuts
2 green onions, chopped
1/4 cup grated carrots
1 TBLS Soy sauce
3 slices fresh ginger chopped or 1 tsp ginger powder
1 tsp. Salt/pepper
8 Cabbage Leaves

Place cabbage leaves in boiling water until limp, 2 minutes
Finely chop water chestnuts, green onion and ginger
Mix with all other ingredients except cabbage leaves
Cut cabbage leaves into 1-1/2" x 3-5" pieces
Spoon small amount of mixture onto each leaf and roll
Steam in double boiler pan for 30 minutes.
Serve with soy sauce

Onion Crackers

100% Whole grain crackers
        (Crunchmaster or Brown Rice Crackers)
1/2 large onion, slice thinly, sauté (low heat) in 2 TBLS
butter, or olive oil, 1/4 cup Marsala wine and 1 clove
chopped garlic for 20 min., until limp
Add another chopped garlic clove, mix all together
Top crackers with onion mixture, and add:
Roasted red pepper, sun-dried tomato/green olives on top

Carrot Cake

1/2 cup xylitol, 1/4 cup coconut sugar or sucanat
1/2 cup sunflower or coconut oil
4 eggs
1 cup oat flour
1 cup blended flour: 1/3 of ea: almond, w/wheat, brown rice
2 tsp baking soda
1 TBLS cinnamon
1/2 tsp nutmeg
1/4 tsp cloves
2 tsp vanilla
1/4 cup coconut and/or almond milk
1/4 cup ground flaxseed (optional)
2 tsp grated orange zest (optional)

3 cups carrot
1/2 cup chopped pineapple

Mix sugars and eggs
Add and mix all ingredients except carrot and pineapple
Stir in carrot and pineapple
Pour into greased and floured pan or muffin tins
325 degrees – 50 min. (muffins: 30 min.)

Apple Cake

2 Apples (dice, do not peel)
1/3 cup fresh pineapple (optional)
2 eggs
1/3 cup Sucanat (or 1/2 banana)
1 tsp vanilla

1 cup blended flour mix
1 TBLS Cinnamon
3/4 tsp baking soda
1/2 tsp salt
1/4 cup oil or alternative milk

Slow cook apples in 1/4 cup water for 15 minutes
Mix eggs, Sucanat, vanilla
Combine all dry ingredients, then add to egg mix
Add apples and mix for a few minutes to combine thoroughly
Mix in oil or milk
Add chopped walnuts (optional)
Pour into greased and floured pan (or parchment liner)
Cook at 325 for about 40 minutes

Custard

6 Eggs
2-1/2 cups coconut or cashew milk
1/4 cup xylitol
1 tsp vanilla
1/2 tsp nutmeg

Mix and divide into cups for baking; put cups into shallow pan of water. Sprinkle nutmeg on top of each cup.
325 degrees, 40 minutes

Pumpkin Flan

5 TBLS Sucanat
1-2/3 cups unsweetened alternative milk
1/3 cup xylitol
5 eggs
2/3 cup pumpkin puree
1/2 tsp vanilla
1/2 tsp cinnamon
1/4 tsp nutmeg

Coat 5 small baking dishes with butter/oil and 1 TBLS Sucanat
Beat Eggs
Add all other ingredients and beat together
Pour into dishes
Put dishes in large pan of water - almost to top of dishes
Bake at 330% for 40 minutes
Let cool for 5-10 minutes; turn over custard onto plates or bowls

Orange Oatmeal Cookies

1 cup butter and/or coconut oil
1/2 cup xylitol
2/3 cup sucanat
2 eggs beaten
3 cups oatmeal
1-1/2 cup flour
        The complete inside of 1 orange (chopped or puréed)
1 tsp grated orange rind
1 tsp vanilla, cinnamon, 1/4 tsp nutmeg

Mix xylitol with 1 TBLS hot water to dissolve (10 min.)
Cream butter/oil and sugars
Add eggs
Add orange and rind. Mix in flours, spices and oatmeal
Drop on greased cookie sheet
Bake at 350 degrees, 12 min.

Lemon Squares

2/3 cup xylitol
1 tsp baking powder
1/4 cup whole wheat flour
3/4 cup lemon juice
1 whole inside of one lemon, mashed
1 TBLS grated, minced lemon peel
4 eggs

Mix xylitol with 1 TBLS hot water to dissolve
Mix all ingredients together
Beat for 1 minute

Make crust

CRUST:

1/3 cup whole wheat flour
1/3 cup oat flour
1/2 cup crushed walnuts
1/2 cup crushed almonds or almond meal
3 TBLS margarine or butter
4 dates, chopped
Mix all together
Spread into pan and cook for 10 minutes
Let cool
Spread lemon mixture on top of crust
Cook another 10 minutes
Let cool, in refrigerator for 1 hour; cut into squares

Chewy Brownie Cookies

3/4 cup coconut oil or: 1/2 cup coconut oil, 1/4 cup raw butter
3/4 cup SUCANAT
1/3 cup xylitol
1 tsp vanilla extract
2 eggs
1 cup whole wheat flour
1/2 cup oat flour
1/2 cup raw unprocessed cacao
1/4 tsp baking soda
1/2 tsp Sea Salt
1 cup chopped walnuts (optional)

Combine oil, Sucanat, xylitol, vanilla
Beat at medium speed
Beat eggs into mixture
Combine flours, cacao, baking soda and salt
Add to wet mixture
Stir in walnuts. Chill in refrigerator for 1 hour
Drop cookie portions onto ungreased cookie sheet
Cook at 380 degrees for 8-9 minutes

Pumpkin Pie

1-3/4 cups plain cooked pumpkin (or canned)
1/2 cup sucanat
1/4 cup xylitol (or all sucanat)
1 TBLS coconut or tapioca flour (mix with sugar)
1/2 tsp sea salt
2 tsp cinnamon
1/2 tsp ginger
1/2 tsp nutmeg
1/2 tsp cloves
4 slightly beaten eggs
1 cup coconut milk (unsweetened in carton)

Combine all ingredients except eggs and milk
Blend eggs and milk, mix with all ingredients until smooth
Pour into pie crust
Bake 400 degrees, 50 minutes

Whipped Cream

1 CAN coconut milk, chilled (*not in the carton; make sure it is plain, without guar gum or other additives*)

1/3 cup powdered sugar (see Chapter 6, *Recipe Replacements*)
1 tsp vanilla
1 tsp lemon juice
1/2 tsp baking soda
1/4 tsp xanthan gum
Carefully open can; solid milk will be on top, water on bottom; carefully spoon out milk solid, and discard water
Beat coconut milk 30 sec.; add all ingredients, Beat till stiff

Pie Crust *(makes 2)*

1-1/3 cups flour blend:
>1/3 sorghum, 1/3 brown rice, 1/3 oat, 1/3 whole wheat
>(options: almond, coconut or amaranth)

1/4 cup coconut oil (cold)
1/4 cup raw butter (cold) (or use all coconut oil)
1/2 tsp xanthan gum (1 w/o using any whole wheat)
1 tsp sea salt
1 TBLS cold water

Put flour, cold butter and salt in food processor; process about 10 seconds until it turns into a coarse meal texture

With processor running, add water through tube

Press dough into pie pan; press down rim of crust
>(not over the rim of the pie tin)

Bake at 350 for 8 minutes
Place in refrigerator to cool before adding filling

After adding filling, cover around rim of pie crust w/strips of aluminum foil to keep from over-browning

You will never have to roll out crusts again.

BREAKFAST

For Waffles, use a flour blend of your choice
I use this flour blend:
1 cup whole wheat
1-1/4 cup oat
1-1/4 cup brown rice
1/2 tsp xanthan gum

Waffles

4 tsp Baking powder
2 tsp cinnamon
1 tsp Salt
6 egg yolks beaten - 6 egg whites beaten stiffly
3 cups alternative milk
3 TBLS apple cider vinegar
1 cup coconut or sunflower oil

Combine vinegar and milk, let sit 10-15 minutes
Combine dry ingredients
Combine egg yolks and milk
Mix together
Stir in oil
Fold in egg whites
(Can be frozen)
Serve with poached eggs, veggie burger, or
spinach cake w/hollandaise

For Pancakes use a flour blend of your choice:
I use this flour blend:
1 cup whole wheat
1/2 cup brown rice
1/2 cup oat

Minnesota Pancakes

4 eggs
2 cups flour blend
2 cups alternative milk
2 TBLS Apple Cider Vinegar
1 tsp sea salt
1 tsp. baking soda
1/2 tsp. cinnamon
4 TBLS sunflower oil

Put vinegar into milk and let sit 5 minutes
Mix dry ingredients, add eggs and mix slowly with fork while
        adding small amounts of milk
Mix until lumps are gone. Mix in oil
Grill on oil-coated surface
(Makes a thinner pancake)
(Can be frozen)
Serve with poached eggs, veggie burger, or
spinach cake w/hollandaise

Pumpkin Pancakes:

Add 2 TBLS cinnamon
1 cup cooked/canned pumpkin

Cinnamon Toast

Sprouted grain bread, toasted
Spread with margarine/butter
Sprinkle with 1/2 - 1 tsp Cinnamon
Spread with 1/2 – 1 tsp raw honey on top

Or Pre-Mix:
Melt 1/2 cup margarine/butter
Add:
2 TBLS cinnamon
2-3 slowly heated, melted raw honey (do not simmer)

Mix all together, and refrigerate

Homemade Berry Sauce

2 cups berries
1/4 cup water
2 tsp fresh lemon juice

Heat ingredients in saucepan on low heat (do not simmer)
Remove from heat
To thicken, mix 1 tsp arrowroot with 1 TBLS water
Mix quickly into heated sauce
Option: mix with 1/3 cup Maple Syrup

Homemade Syrup

1 cup Sucanat or Coconut sugar
2/3 cup water
Lightly heat until Sucanat is dissolved (do not simmer)

(Or simply use coconut nectar out of the jar)

French Toast

8 slices of sprouted grain bread
5-6 large eggs
1/2 cup alternative milk
2 tsp cinnamon
1-1/2 cups fresh or frozen (thawed) berries, whole or mashed

Toast the bread lightly, and let cool; Cut off crust (optional)
Mix eggs, milk and cinnamon in shallow rectangle baking pan
Soak bread slices, both sides, in egg mixture until drenched

Prepare another shallow rectangle pan
        w/parchment paper on bottom
Place 4 soaked slices in pan; spread berries on top of bread
Place remaining bread slices on top of berries (like a sandwich)
Cover pan with foil; Bake in oven for 30 min. at 295 degrees
When ready, top with butter and real maple syrup

EGGS

Always slow-cook eggs on the lowest burner setting.

Use GREEN pans only (these are non-teflon, ceramic coated pans, labeled as a green product.)

Here is my technique for cooking eggs the healthy way:
1. Prepare the vegetables you'd like to have with your eggs.
2. Put them in a *green* skillet with 1 TBLS water. (Or just eat them raw by adding after the eggs cook).
3. Cover and bring temperature up for a few seconds to get the heat started.
4. Lower to the lowest setting on the stove.
5. Cook for 2 minutes then turn off.
6. Let sit for 5 minutes; It will continue cooking on its own.
7. This will soften and not overcook the vegetables.
8. Spread one TBLS olive oil on the bottom of the pan, leaving in the vegetables.
9. Break eggs into the pan.
10. Cover and turn the burner to the lowest setting once again.
11. Eggs will take from 9 to 12 minutes to slow cook to perfection, sunnyside up;
    Do not turn over.

Order of best in nutritional quality:
Poached
Soft Boiled
Slow-Fried (sunnyside up only; when covered, eggs cook like over-easy)
Hard Boiled
Scrambled

To Scramble Eggs:

Coat bottom of pan with 2 TBLS oil or butter, and warm
Add eggs to pan
Stir eggs w/spatula; as it starts to cook, stir very fast,
Remove from heat and keep stirring
Return it to heat, and stir again, until they are cooked through
   (milk, butter or cheese are unnecessary for scrambled eggs or omelets)

Various vegetables can be added:

Chopped green onions	Tomatoes
Sliced sweet onion	Sun-Dried Tomatoes
Spinach	Mushrooms
Green pepper	Artichoke hearts
Green chiles	Zucchini

Cover pan, and cook on lowest flame possible
Check frequently, and stir until done; do not overcook

Italian Eggs

Chop sweet or green onions
Soften
Add 1 TBLS sun-dried tomatoes (per serving)
Break eggs into pan
Salt and pepper
Cover and cook on lowest flame for 5-10 min.
Add sun-dried tomatoes to eggs
Cover and cook until eggs are done

Green Eggs

With Spinach, grated zucchini, green onion, artichokes

Mexican Eggs

Anaheim chiles and onion, chopped
Top with cilantro and salsa; optional sliced avocado

Mediterranean Eggs

Cut 2 hard boiled eggs into quarters; Add tomato chunks, onion chunks, cucumber chunks, (option: crumbled raw goat cheese), Greek olives, 1 tsp. olive oil, 1 TBLS lemon juice, sprinkle with black pepper (option: garbanzo beans) Toss and eat

Eggs Foo Yung

4 Eggs (for two)
2 cups fresh packaged bean sprouts and/or chopped bok choy
1/3 cup sliced onions
1/3 cup cut-up or sliced mushrooms
2 cloves freshly chopped garlic
Wheat-free soy sauce (Tamari, San-J brand)
1 TBLS expeller-pressed oil

Lightly steam vegetables in 1 TBLS water, covered 5 minutes.

Add 2 TBLS oil to coat pan, scramble eggs w/vegetables on low heat
When eggs are half done, mix in soy sauce and garlic
Stir on low heat until eggs are done

(Traditional egg foo yong is a browned egg patty; these eggs eliminate the browning)

Eggs w/Mushrooms & Peppers

Sliced mushrooms
Pre-prepared roasted sliced green, yellow, red peppers, onion

Slice all peppers and onions, add garlic, Greek olives, and 1 TBLS olive oil, roast in oven (350 degrees) for 30 minutes, turning frequently; this mixture can be on hand for the week to use on sandwiches, breakfast eggs or dinner side dish any time during the week.

REFERENCES

"Achievements in Public Health, 1900-1999: Decline in Deaths from Heart Disease and Stroke – United States, 1900-1999." 1999. Centers for the Disease Control and Prevention. *Morbidity and Mortality Weekly Report.*

Ament, M. 2008. "Why refined sugar is the most dangerous 'food' you can eat." *SelfGrowth.com.*

Anderson, R.N. "Deaths: Leading causes for 2000". *National Vital Statistics Reports NVSS*, CDC, Volume 50, Number 16. Division of Vital Statistics.

Axe, J. 2010. "Why you should avoid pork". *Maximize Your Health.* http://www.draxe.com/why-you-should-avoid-pork/.

Bible Verses About Eating Pork. The Official King James Bible Online. N.a. http://www.kingjamesbibleonline.org/Bible-Verses-About-Eating-Pork/

Bohne, M., Halloran, J. 2012. "Meat on drugs." *Consumer Reports.*

Bowden, J. 2007. *The 150 Healthiest Foods on Earth.* Beverly, MA: Fair Winds Press.

"Breakfast, blood glucose, and cognition." Benton, D, Parker, P.Y. *American Journal of Clinical Nutrition.* 1998

Brown, Dr. S, & Trivieri, Jr., L. 2006. *The Acid Alkaline Food Guide.* New York: Square One Publishers.

Causes, risk factors, and prevention topics. 2012. The American Cancer Society. http://www.cancer.org/Cancer/BreastCancer/ DetailedGuide/breast-cancer-risk-factors

Cutler, DC, E. 2005. *Micro Miracles.* New York: Rodale Books.

Davis, M.S., et al. 2005. "Cold weather exercise and airway cytokine expression." American Physiological Society. Journal of Applied Physiology. jap.physiology.org.

Devries, D. *How does a freezer work?* eHow.com.

A Diner's Guide to Health and Nutrition Claims on Restaurant Menus. 1997. CSPI Reports. Centre for Science in the Public Interest. Canada.

Dong, F.M. 2009. "The nutritional value of shellfish". *University of Illinois.* http://wsg.washington.edu/communications/online/ shellfishnutrition_09.pdf

Enig, M.G., Fallon, S. 2000. "The Skinny on Fats." Weston A. Price Foundation.

"Executive summary from the report: Analysis of adverse reactions to monosodium glutamate (MSG)." *Center for Food Safety and Applied Nutrition, Food and Drug Administration.* 1995. jn.nutrition.org

Fallon, S., Enig, M.G. 2002. "The Great Con-Ola". *Weston A. Price Foundation* 21:49.

Fallon, S. 2008. "The ploy of soy." *Nourished Magazine.*

Fallon, S., and Enig, M., Ph.D. 1995. *Health Freedom News.*

Fassa, P. 2009. *Confronting Salt Confusion.* Natural News.

"Feeding Farmed Salmon". *Pure Salmon Campaign.* http://www.puresalmon.org

Gagnon, M., Freudenberg, N. 2012. "Slowing Down Fast Food." City University of New York School of Public Health at Hunter College and Corporate Accountability International. Boston, MA. *Natural Resources Defense Council (NRDC):* NY.

Galloway, J. H. 1989. *The sugar cane industry. An historical geography from its origins to 1914.* Cambridge.

Ganmaa, D., Sato, A. 2005. "Milk from Pregnant Cows Is Responsible for the Development of Breast, Ovarian and Corpus Uteri Cancers", Adapted from: "The Possible Role of Female Sex Hormones in Milk from Pregnant Cows in the Development of Breast, Ovarian and Corpus Uteri Cancers". *Medical Hypotheses* 2005; 65 (6): 1028-37.

Haas, E.M., Levin, B. 2006. *Staying Healthy with Nutrition.* Berkeley: Celestial Arts.

Haas, M.D., E. 2004. *The New Detox Diet.* Berkeley: Celestial Arts.

History of medicine 1800-1850. n.d. Wellness Directory of Minnesota. http://www.mnwelldir.org/docs/history/history03.htm.

Holford, P. 2004. *The New Optimum Nutrition Bible.* Berkeley: Crossing Press

How does a freezer work? WiseGEEK.org. http://www.wisegeek.org/how-does-a-refrigerator-work.htm

Houlihan, J., et. al. 2003. "Teflon toxicosis: EWG finds heated Teflon pans can turn toxic faster than DuPont claims". http://www.ewg.org/research/canaries-kitchen

How Nutritious Are Potatoes? 2004. Baylor College of Medicine. http://www.bcm.edu/cnrc/consumer/archives/potatoe.htm

Hybarger, C. 2007. "Cooking in the 1800s. When dinner wasn't quick and easy." http://ncpedia.org/culture/food/cooking-in-the-1800s

Jones, D.S. 2006. "The persistence of American Indian health disparities". American Journal of Public Health. http://www.ncbi.nlm.nih.gov/pmc/articles/PMC1698152/

Kliment, F. 2002. *The Acid Alkaline Balance Diet.* New York: McGraw Hill.

"Love Is The Doctor L'Amour Medecin, Moliere 1622-1673". *Pearson Education.* Pearson Literature. n.d.

Lundell, D., Nordstrom, T.R. 2007. *The Cure for Heart Disease: Truth Will Save a Nation*, Scottsdale, AZ: Heart Surgeons Health Plan.

Mäkinen, K.K. 1976. "Long-term tolerance of healthy human subjects to high amounts of xylitol and fructose: general and biochemical findings." Int Z Vitam Ernahrungsforsch Beih. 15:92-104.

Mattila, P., Hellstrom, J. 2006. "Phenolic acids in potatoes, vegetables, and some of their products". MTT Agrifood Research Finland, *Biotechnology and Food Research*, ET-talo, FIN-31600.

Mihesuah, D.A. n.a. "American Indian Health and Diet Project." The University of Kansas. Humanities and Western Civilization. http://www.aihd.ku.edu/

Mihesuah, D.A., et al. 2005. "Health problems: History of declining health." "Recovering our ancestors' gardens: Indigenous recipes and guides to diet and fitness". *University of Nebraska Press.* http://www.aihd.ku.edu/health/history_declining_health.html

Montaigne, F. 2003. "Everybody loves Atlantic salmon". *National Geographic Magazine.*

Müller, M.J., et al. 1996. Institute for Clinical & Experimental Surgery, University of Saarland, Homburg/Saar, Germany. *Free Radic Biol Med.*

Murray, M.T., Pizzorno, J., 2012. *The Encyclopedia of Natural Medicine.* New York: Atria.

Nagel, R. 2008. "Agave Nectar, the High Fructose Health Food Fraud." Naturalnews.com

Nuts for the heart. n.a. Harvard School of Public Health. http://www.hsph.harvard.edu/nutritionsource/nuts-for-the-heart/

Nagel, R. 2008. "Agave nectar, the high fructose health food fraud." *www.naturalnews.com.*

Packer, L, Colman, C. 1999. *The Antioxidant Miracle.* New York: John Wiley & Sons, Inc.

Ravnskov, U. 2009. *Fat and Cholesterol are Good for You.* Calgary: GB Publishing.

"Refined-cereal intake and risk of selected cancers in Italy". *The American Journal of Clinical Nutrition.* 1999. 1–3.

Reinagel, M. 2006. *The Inflammation Free Diet Plan.* New York: McGraw Hill.

Salazar, M.J. 2005. "Effect of an Avocado Oil-Rich Diet Over an Angiotensin II-Induced Blood Pressure Response". *Journal of Ethnopharmacology.*

Séralini, G., et al. 2012. "Long term toxicity of a Roundup herbicide and a Roundup-tolerant genetically modified maize." *Food and Chemical Toxicology.* Volume 50, Issue 11, Pages 4221–4231.

Shier, D., Butler, J., Lewis, R. 2006. *Hole's Essentials of Human Anatomy and Physiology.* New York: McGraw-Hill.

Shinya, MD, H. 2008. *The Enzyme Factor.* Canada: Council Oak Books.

Smythies, J.R. 1998. *Every Person's Guide to Antioxidants.* New Jersey: Rutgers University Press.

Somer, E. 2000. "Does Chinese Food Give You a Headache?" *WebMD Health News.*

Sompayrac, L. 2008. *How the Immune System Works.* Malden, MA: Blackwell Publishing

Taubes, G. 2008. *Good Calories, Bad Calories: Fats, Carbs, and the Controversial Science of Diet and Health.* New York: Anchor.

Thibodeau, G.A., Patton, K.T. 2008. *Structure & Function of the Body.* St. Louis: Mosby Elsevier.

Thomas, P. 2008. *What's In This Stuff? The Hidden Toxins in Everyday Products and What You Can Do About Them.* New York: Perigee Trade.

"Triclosan and triclocarban". 2011. *Natural Resources Defense Council.* http://www.nrdc.org/living/chemicalindex/triclosan.asp

"Triglycerides and Cardiovascular Disease". *American Heart Association.* AHA Scientific Statement. http://circ.ahajournals.org/content/123/20/2292.long

Verwymeren, A. 2011. "Alternatives to plastic wrap". http://www.networx.com/article/alternatives-to-plastic-wrap

Wahaidi, V.Y. 2005. "The systemic inflammatory response to dental plaque." *Indiana University-Purdue University Indianapolis IUPUI, Dentistry School Theses and Dissertations.* https://scholarworks.iupui.edu/handle/1805/2086

Walton, A.G. 2012. "How much sugar are Americans eating?" http://www.Forbes.com/sites/alicegwalton

Welshons, W., et. al. 2006. *Large Effects from Small Exposures. III. Endocrine Mechanisms Mediating Effects of Bisphenol A at Levels of Human Exposure.* University of Missouri-Columbia.

"*Willow Bark.*" n.d. University of Maryland Medical Center. http://www.umm.edu/altmed/articles/willow-bark-000281.htm

Woolfe, J.A. 1987. *The Potato in the Human Diet.* Cambridge: Cambridge University Press.

Young, R. O., Young, S. R. 2010. *The pH Miracle: Balance your Diet, Reclaim Your Health*. New York: Warner Books.

Zheng, W., Lee, S.A. "Well-done meat intake, heterocyclic amine exposure, and cancer risk." Vanderbilt-Ingram Cancer Center, Vanderbilt University School of Medicine.

INDEX

RECIPE INDEX

Recommended Professional Advocates
of Nutrition To Follow

Dr. Mark Hyman   http://drhyman.com/

Dr. John McDougall   http://www.drmcdougall.com/

Dr. Dean Ornish   http://www.ornishspectrum.com/

Dr. Joel Fuhrman   http://www.drfuhrman.com/

Dr. Michael Murray   http://doctormurray.com/

Dr. Frank Lipman   http://www.drfranklipman.com/

Dr. Joseph Mercola, D.O.   http://www.mercola.com/

Byron Richards, C.N.   http://www.byronrichards.com/

Dr. Josh Axe, D.C., CNS   http://www.draxe.com/

Institute of Functional Medicine

http://www.functionalmedicine.org/

Recommended Websites
Focused on Health & Nutrition

Science Daily   http://www.sciencedaily.com/

What's In This Stuff   http://www.whatsinthisstuff.com/

NutritionData   http://nutritiondata.self.com/

Natural News   http://www.naturalnews.com/

Earth Clinic   http://www.earthclinic.com/

Vitacost Supplements and Health Food

http://www.vitacost.com

iHerb Supplements and Health Food

http://www.iherb.com

Pure Formulas Supplements

http://www.pureformulas.com

FDA Recalls/Safety Alerts

http://www.fda.gov/safety/recalls/default.htm

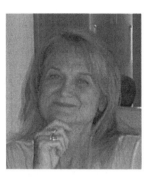

Linda Larrowe Bergersen, MS, Board Certified Holistic Nutritionist, follows the *Functional Medicine* agenda of treating the person, and not just the symptoms. She treats individuals through a specialized regimen, and conducts seminars on nutrition. Her articles can be found on HuffingtonPost.com and the SDGLN network. She holds an M.S. in holistic nutrition, a B.A. in communications, and lives in Palm Springs, CA, with her husband.

Made in the USA
San Bernardino, CA
28 March 2014